PHARMACOGENOMICS
An Approach to New Drug Development

by

Dr. Chiranjib Chakraborty

Manager-Biotechnology (R&D), Glenmark Laboratories, Mumbai;
(Previously—Research Scientist, Biotechnology,
Macleods Pharmaceuticals Ltd., Mumbai;
Lecturer, Deaprtment of Industrial Fish and Fishery, Burdwan Raj College,
Burdwan, West Bengal, India)

&

Dr. Atanu Bhattacharyya

Reader, Department of Zoology,
Vidyasagar College for Women, Kolkata, West Bengal, India.
(Previously—Assistant Director, West Bengal State Sericulture,
Small Scale Industry, West Bengal, India)

BIOTECH

2013

BIOTECH BOOKS®

2013
ISBN 81-7622-105-8

Published by : **BIOTECH BOOKS**
1123/74, Tri Nagar,
Delhi - 110 035
Phone: 27382765
e-mail: biotechbooks@yahoo.co.in

Showroom : 4762-63/23, Ansari Road, Darya Ganj,
New Delhi - 110 002
Phone: 23245578, 23244987

Laser Typesetting : **Classic Computer Services**
Delhi - 110 035

Printed at : **Chawla Offset Printers**
Delhi - 110 052

PRINTED IN INDIA

Preface

The era of molecular medicine has arrived. The journey of molecular medicine was started about 50 years ago when James Watson and Francies Crick discovered the structure of DNA. Molecular medicine involves the applications of Biotechnology and Bioinformatics. These new drugs that facilitated by the Biotechnology and Bioinformatics will replace medications due to competition from generic drugs in the next five years as patents run out. The microarray technology is the future direction of diagnosis. These development in science and medicine are so far-reaching that the words of celebrated C S Lewis "Each new power won by man is a power over man as well" could well apply to the power of Biotechnology and Bioinformatics for new drug development.

At present, life expectancy has increased day by day by these new drugs. In this situation, we think, this book will be a landmark for the student, researchers as well as professional in various spheres of pharmaceutical industry. It is a compilation of different aspects like molecular engineering of protein for new drug, DNA chips, genomic image processing for development of new drugs, DNA vaccination, combo-vaccination, gene therapy and some other modern topics.

In the preparation of manuscripts, help has been taken from various materials, which has been duly acknowledged in the text. Every effort has been made to properly acknowledge the various source of information included in the script. Criticisms and suggestions are always welcome from the readers.

This is a first comprehensive account that deals with different aspects of modern Biotechnological and Bio-informational research for new drugs. We sincerely hope that this issue will be an important source of information on modern Biotechnological and Bio-informational research for new drug discovery.

Dr. Chiranjib Chakraborty
Dr. Atanu Bhattacharyya

Contents

CHAPTER 1

DNA Chips Technology for Implementation of Genomic Drugs

Introduction

The DNA chips known as Gene Chip, consist of a tiny computer chip, which contents genetic information as well as electric sensors. The sensors can be tested for determination of various genetic diseases. The result is displayed on a computer screen from which new drug can be recommended to ameliorate those genetic diseases. This article will discuss how a DNA chip could be designed for implementation of new genomic drugs in modern medicine industry.

It is widely believed that thousand of genes and their products (*i.e.* RNA and proteins) in a given living organism function in a complicated and orchestrated manner that creates the mystery of life. However, traditional methods in molecular biology generally work on a "one gene in one experiment" basis which means that the throughput is very limited and the "whole picture" of gene function is difficult to obtain. Several years back, a new technology, called DNA microarray, had attracted tremendous interests among biologists. This technology promises to monitor the whole genome on a single chips (called DNA chips) so that researcher can have a better picture of the interactions among thousands of genes simultaneously (1,2,3).

An array is an orderly arrangement of samples. It provides a medium for matching known and unknown DNA samples based on base-ɪ airing rules and automating the process of identifying the unknowr ›. An array experiment can make use of common assay systems ɩuch as microplates or standard blotting membranes, and can be created by hand or make use of robotics to deposit the sample (4). In general, arrays are described as *macroarrays* or *microarrays*, the difference being the size of the sample spots. Macroarrays contain sample spot that sizes of about 300 microns or larger and can be easily imaged by existing gel and blot scanners.

The sample spot sizes in microarray are typically less than 200 microns in diameter and these arrays usually contains thousands of spots (5,6). Here, array generally refers to microarrays.

The Gene Chip contents genetic information as well as electric sensors. The sensors can be tested for genetic diseases in a way. Each sport on the chip will detect matching stands. Attaching small fluorescent molecules to the stands can be making them easily seen upon laser scanning. The DNA fragments can be heated and mixed with reagents to show the genetic code or the DNA can be squirted on the chip, where the sample is compared with normal DNA stand. The mismatches are highlighted, and the diseased one could be determined. This result is displayed on a computer screen from which new drug can be implemented for genetic diseases. This chapter will discuss how a DNA chip will be designed for implementation of new genomic drugs.

Array Types Variants of the DNA Microarray Technology

There are two variants of the DNA microarray technology, in terms of the property of arrayed DNA sequence with known identity: Complete or partial cDNA and Oligonucleotides or DNA fragments. Complete or partial cDNA (approximately 500-5,000 nucleotide beases long) arrays are generally used for relative gene expression analysis of two or more samples (7), however, oligonucleotide based arrays may also be used for these studies. Probe cDNA (500-5,000 bases) is immobilized to a solid surface such as glass using robot spotting and exposed to a set of targets either separately or in a mixture. This method, "traditionally" called DNA microarray, is widely considered as developed at Stanford University (8).

Oligonucleotides or DNA fragments (approximately 20-25 nucleotide bases) arrays are frequently used in gene typing experiments. The sequences of alternate gene forms may be included for detection of mutations or normal variants (polymorphisms). An array of oligonucleotide (20-25-mer oligos) or peptide nucleic acid (PNA) probes is synthesized either *in situ* (on-chip) or by conventional synthesis followed by on-chip immobilization. The array is exposed to labelled sample DNA, hybridized, and the identity/abundance of complementary sequences are determined. This method, "historically" called DNA chips, was developed at Affymetrix, Inc., (which sells its products under the 'Gene Chip' trademark), USA.

Design of A DNA Microarray System

DNA microarrays typically consist of thousands of immobilized DNA sequences present on a miniaturized surface the size of a business card or less. Arrays are used to analyze a sample for the presence of gene variations or mutations (genotyping), or for patterns of gene expression, performing the equivalent of ca. 5,000 to 10,000 individual "test tube" experiments in approximately two days of time.

Microarrays require specialized robotics and imaging equipment that generally are not commercially available as a complete system. DNA microarray, or DNA chips are fabricated by these high-speed robotics, generally on glass but sometimes on nylon substrates, for which probes (According to B. Phimister (1999) (9) – a "probe" is the tethered nucleic acid with known sequence, whereas a "target" is the free nucleic acid sample whose identity/abundance is being detected) with known identity are used to determine complementary binding, thus allowing massively parallel gene expression and gene discovery studies, An experiment with a single DNA chip can provide researchers information on thousands of genes simultaneously – a dramatic increase in throughput.

Alterations in gene expression patterns (10) or in a DNA sequence can have profound effects on biological functions. These variations in gene expression are at the core of altered physiologic and pathologic processes. DNA array technology provides rapid and cost-effective methods of identifying gene expression and genetic variations.

Robotic technology (11) is employed in the preparation of most arrays. The DNA sequences are bound to a surface such as a nylon membrane or glass slide at precisely defined locations on a grid. Using an alternate method, some arrays are produced using laser lithographic processes and are referred to as biochips or gene chips.

There are several steps in the design and implementation of a DNA microarray experiment. Many strategies have been investigated at each of these steps. There are – (1) DNA types; (2) Chip fabrication; (3) Sample preparation; (4) Assay; (5) Readout and (6) Software (informatics) which is describe in Table 1.1.

TABLE 1.1: Steps in the Design and Implementation of a DNA Microarray Experiment

Steps for the Design and Implementation of DNA Chips	*Description*
DNA types *i.e.* Probe (cDNA/oligo with known identity)	Small oligos, cDNAs, chromosome, etc.
Chip fabrication (Putting probes on the chip)	Photolighography, pipette, drop-touch, piezoelectric (ink-jet), electric etc.
Target (fluorecently labelled sample)	RNA, (mRNA →) cDNA
Assay	Hybridization, long, short, ligase, base addition, electric, MS, electrophoresis, fluocytometry, PCR-DIRECT, TaqMan, etc.
Readout	Fluorescence, probeless (conductance, MS, electrophoresis), electronic etc.
Informatics	Robotics control, Image processing, DBMS, WWW, bioinformatics, data mining and visualization.

DNA samples are prepared from the cells or tissues of interest. For genotyping analysis, the sample is genomic DNA. For expression analysis, the sample is cDNA, DNA copies of RNA. The DNA samples are tagged with a radioactive or flourescent label and applied to the array. Single-stranded DNA will bind to a complementary strand of DNA. At positions on the array where the immobilized DNA recognizes a complementary DNA in the sample, binding or hybridization occurs. The labelled sample DNA marks the exact position on the array where binding occurs, allowing automatic detection. The output consists of a list of hybridization events, indicating the presence or the relative abundance of specific DNA sequences that are present in the sample.

Oligonucleotide synthesis is carried out on a glass surface (*"in silico"*), using photolithography or maskless mirrors (Micromirrors). In the first case, each array requires a set of photolithographic masks. Precursors are photosensitive hydroxyl-protected deoxynucleotides, which are tethered at the 5′ end and reactive at the 3′-OH end after light activation. Synthesis of oligonucleotides is brought about by light-induced deprotection and masking areas of synthesis. The oligonucleotide products constitute immobile phase DNA (12) (Fig. 1.1). The degree of hybridization is assessed by monitoring fluorescent emission (13) using laser excitation that is focussed at the interface between the surface of the glass slide (immobile phase) and the solution (mobile phase). Imaging methods typically involve a dedicated confocal scanning device. A 2-dimensional image is created, with each spot being identified by its coordinates on the microarray (rink to an image). Once images are obtained into digitized form, they are transferred to a separate workstation for analysis. A variety of software programs are being developed to accomplish the analysis efficiently.

Hybridization is typically quantified by imaging of the fluorescent signals using software specifically designed for this purpose. Signals are measured as absolute intensities for a given target, or as ratios of two probes with different fluorescent labels representing two separate treatments to be compared or with one probe as an internal control. Background is subtracted by different methods, depending on the software used. The ratio of two signals provides relative response ratios rather than an estimate of an absolute signal. (10,14,15)

The objective of the microarray image analysis is to extract probe intensities or ratios at each cDNA target location, and then cross-link printed clone target information so that biologists can easily interpret the outcomes and perform further high-level analysis. However, the microarray image sources are not only from one print-mode, *i.e.*, number of printing tip (16) or one hybridization method, *i.e.*, fluorescent or radioactive probe.

FIGURE 1.1: Flowchart of DNA Microarray Protocols from Cultured Human Cells

Preparation of total RNA from cultural human cells.

↓

Preparation of polyA + mRNA from total human RNA.

↓

Amplification and purification of cDNAs for microarray manufacture.

↓

Microarray manufacture and processing.

↓

Generating control mRNAs by *in vitro* transcription.

↓

Generating fluorescent cDNA controls by linear PCR.

↓

Preparation of fluorescent probes from total human mRNA.

↓

cDNA microarray hybridization and washing.

↓

Gene expression analysis with microarrays.

↓

Mutation detection with oligonucleotide microarrays.

For this particular image example, all array of cDNAs was hybridized with a red fluor-tagged sample and green fluor-tagged sample, and then monochrome images of the fluorescent intensity were combined by placing each image into the appropriate color channel of the RGB color image. In this experiment, there were a total of 1,344 cDNA targets (printed from fourteen 96-well plates) using four print-tips, By defining the print-mode, the software can track the cDNA targets on this and the other array, and map them back to their original plate position.

FIGURE 1.2: Flowchart of Experimental Protocols DNA Microarray Preparation in General

DNA Sample Preparation

↓

Slide Preparation (Poly-l-Lysine Coating of Slides).

↓

Directions for Printing Arrays

↓

Nucleic Acid Preparation (Human Fast Track mRNA Isolation)

↓

Nucleic Acid Labelling Reverse Transcription using Cy3- and Cy5-dUTP: (Yeast, Human, *E. Coli*)

↓

Array Post Processing

↓

Array Hybridization Scanning Microarrays

↓

Data Processing

↓

Miscellaneous (Cy dye HPLC Purification and Genomic Design)

A set of software tools is being developed. The tool suite is a collection of IP Lab extensions for the Macintosh computer (IP Lab is an image processing package by Scalytics). Some of tools include:

1. Load SKN, which loads images from the NIH scanner or other scanning instruments.
2. Align Array, which aligns two images in case the images from red and green channels were scanned separately.
3. DeArray, which is the central processing tool controlling most of image processing tasks, including target segmentation, background intensity, estimation and probable intensity extraction.

4. Target locator, which reports target information, refines statistics, and performs some image enhancement tasks. The development of the Array Suite is a continuous process, along with the perfection of the microarray technology and the progress or various applications of the technology.

Discussion

Very often, we experience a number of enigmatic aspects governing the biomolecular functions in the living systems, naturally one can question why some drugs work better in some patients than in others? And why some drugs may even be highly toxic to certain patients? The modified definition must be Pharmacogenomics, is the hybridization of functional genomics and molecular pharmacology (17). The goal of pharmacogenomics is to find correlations between therapeutic responses to drugs and genetic profiles of patients (18).

The traditional approach to drug discovery involved previously known target enzymes and pathways, which were screened for structure/function optimization. A barrier to effective drug discovery was the limited number of target proteins (about 500 total). With the advent of molecular biology and gene cloning, human proteins were provided that allowed manipulations of dangerous molecules by site directed mutagenesis.

The human genome project could potentially provide thousands of new targets as the functional roles of newly identified genes become clear (19). But what is the association of proteins with disease? And how are individual genotypes, proteins and drugs to be related? It is now possible to map the location of a genetic variation that corresponds with a phenotype in order to identify genes involved in disease resistance. Through characterization of genomic responses to disease in humans and other experimented animals, genes may be discovered for new drug development. According to Marton *et al.* (20) DNA microarrays drug target validation and identification of secondary drug, target effects can be performed. A number of microarray laboratories have given thought to formulating such a standard. Ideally, such a standard would provide modest signals for every human gene, so that expression of any gene in the experimental probe could be assigned a highly reliable ratio value. Efforts to produce such a reference standard are underway.

Potentially, diagnostic chips can be produced for medical evaluation, forensics and in the arena of new genomic drug development.

Thus, we can surmise that in DNA chips technology relating to 'microarray development' for identifying genetic drugs in the process of ameliorating a number of dreadful diseases. And the technology would become a harbinger in developing modern medicine in the coming millennium.

References

1. Gwynne, P. and Page, G. (1999). Microarray analysis the next revolution in molecular biology. *Science*. 8: 1871-1896.
2. Scherf, U., Ross, D.T., Waltham, M., Smith, L.H., Lee, J.K., Tanabe, L., Kohn, K.W., Reinhold, W.C., Mayers, T.G., Andrews, D.T., Scudiero, D.A., Eisen, M.B., Sausville, E.A., Pommier, Y., Botstein, D., Sinclair, B. (1999). Everything's Great When it Sits on a Chip: A bright future for DNA arrays. *The Scientist*, 13(11): 18-20.
3. Lemieu, B., Aharoni, A., and M. Schena. (1998). Overview of DNA chip technology. *Molecular Breeding*, 4: 277-289.
4. Cortese, J.D. (2000b). The array of today: Biomolecule arrays become the 21st century's test tube. *The Scientist*, 14(17): 25.
5. Service, R.F. (1998a). Microchip arrays put DNA on the spot. *Science*, 282(5388): 396-399.
6. Service, R.F. (1998b). Coming spon: The pocket DNA sequencer. *Science*, 282(5388): 399-401.
7. Pollack, J.R., Perou, C.M., Alizadeh, A.A., Eisen, M.B., Pergamenschikov, A., Williams, C.F., Jeffrey, S.S., Botstein, D., Brown, P.O. (Standford) (1999). Genome-wide analysis DNA copy-number changes using cDNA microarray. *Nat. Genet.*, 23(1): 41-46.
8. Ekins, R. and Chu, F.W. (1999). Microarrays: Their origins and applications. *Trends in Biotechnology*, 17: 217-218.
9. Philllister, B. (1999). An over view of database on DNA-Chips technology. *Nature Genetics*, 22: 46-52.
10. Lockhart, D.J. and E.A. Winzeler (2000). Genomics, gene expression and DNA arrays, *Nature*, 405(6788): 827-836.

11. Cortese, J.D. (2000a). Array of options: Instrumentation to exploint the DNA microarray explosion. *The Scientist*, 29, 14(11): 26.

12. Kane, M.D., Jathoe, T.A., Stumpf, C.R., Lu, J., Thomas, J.D., Madore, S.J. (2000). Assessment of the sensitivity and specificity of oligonucleotide (50mer) micorarrays. *Nucleic Acids Res.*, 28(22): 4552-4557.

13. Shaon, D., Smith, S.J. and Brown, P.O. (1996) (Stanford). A DNA microarray system for analyzing complex DNA samples using two-color fluorescent proble hybridization. *Genomic Res.*, 6(7): 639-645.

14. Reichert, J. (2000). Chip-Based optical detection of DNA hybridization by means of Nanobead labeling. *Anal. Chem.*, 72(24): 6025-6029.

15. Reinke, V., Smith, H.E., Nance, J., Wang, J., Van Doren, C., Begley, R., Jones, S.J., Davis, E.B., Scherer, S., Ward, S., Kim, S.K. (2000). A global profile of germline gene expression in *C. elegans*. *Mol. Cell.*, 6(3): 605-616.

16. MacBeath, G. and S.L. Schreiber. (2000). Printing proteins as microarrays for high-throughput function determination. *Science*, 8: 289(5485): 1760-1763.

17. Housman, D. and Ledley, F. (1998). Why pharmacogenomics? Why now? *Nature Biotechnology*, 16(6): 492-493.

18. Afshari, C.A., Nuwaysir, E.F. and Barrett, J.C. (NIEHS) (1999). Application of complementary DNA microarray technology to carcinogen identification, toxicology, and drug safety evaluation. *Cancer Res.*, 59(19): 4759-4760.

19. Marton, M.J., DeRisi, J.L., Bennett, H.A., Iyer, V.R., Meyer, M.R., Roberts, C.J., Stoughton, R., Burchard, S., Slade, D., Dai, H., Bassett, D.E. Jr., Hartwell, L.H. Brown, P.O., Friend, S.H. (Rosetta/Stanford) (1998). Drug target validation and identification of secondary drug target effects using DNA microarrays. *Nat. Med.*, 4(11): 1293-1301.

20. Brow, P.O. and Weinstein, J.N. (2000). A gene expression database for the molecular pharmacology of cancer. *Nat. Genet.*, 24(3) 236-244.

CHAPTER 2

NEW DNA VACCINES Another Milestone for Pharmaceutical Industry

Introduction

DNA-mediated immunization, called DNA vaccination, are found to be safer and cheaper and expected to change the entire scenario of vaccination. This chapter rcviews an outlook of DNA vaccination, simplified methodology of DNA vaccination, CTL responses and DNA vaccination. plasmid DNA as vector for DNA vaccination, hepatitis B surface antigen and DNA vaccination, HbsAg particles as carriers of heterologous epitopes, status of oral DNA vaccination and our view for some important points of DNA vaccination.

Proteins and proteinaceous substances have been used for immunization previously. Even when polysaccharides or small organic molecules were used, they were coupled to carrier proteins. The reason is the immune system requires peptide epitopes to activate T cells to provide the helper functions necessary for the H2est and most durable immune responses. Protein-based immunization is thus at the basis of the truism, vaccination is not always an overwhelming success, for many reasons. For example, the vaccine to hepatitis B virus comprising either the purified or the incidence of hepatitis B since its introduction in the early 1980's (1). It is thought that the incidence of hepatitis B, which is blood-borne, has probably decreased in certain populations more as a result of safe-sex practices in the wake of the emerging AIDS epidemic although this situation is also due to low vaccine coverage and new methods for vaccine development are nonetheless of great interest. .

Scientific progress is founded – more frequently than imagined – on methodological innovation. Thus, when the occasional revolution in vaccine methodology comes along, it is worth taking a serious look. New methods, in the hands of creative investigators, lead to new experimental approaches which give rise to new concepts and, occasionally, produce shifts in paradigms. Such a methodological leap would appear to have occurred with the advent of DNA-mediated immunization, now colloquially known as DNA vaccines (2). This chapter is an total outlook on DNA vaccination, simplified methodology of DNA vaccination, CTL responses and DNA vaccination, plasmid DNA as vector for DNA vaccination, hepatitis B surface antigen and DNA vaccination, HBsAg particles as carriers of heterologous epitopes, status of oral DNA vaccination and our view for some important points of DNA vaccination.

An Outlook of DNA Vaccines

DNA vaccine technology is Showing increasing promise in the treatment of human diseases, and should offer immunization that are both safer and cheaper than conventional vaccines, according to a new consensus report released by the American Academy of Microbiology.

It suggests that DNA vaccination may revolutionize the practice of human immunization. Recent results obtained from DNA-vaccine testing in animal models suggest that this new technology may revolutionize the vaccination of human and it induce immune responses against diarrhoea-causing viruses, malarial parasites and tuberculosis concluded by Harriet Robinson and his co-authors of Emory University, USA (6).

Conventional vaccines have prevented many millions of cases of killer diseases such as small pox and polio. But some pathogens, such as malaria, have proven to be a considerable challenge to vaccine developers. It is in such cases that DNA vaccines may prove useful. Indeed, a promising DNA vaccine candidate has been developed for malaria, DNA vaccines are also currently being developed for over I5 other human illnesses including AIDS, herpes, tuberculosis and rotavirus, a common cause of childhood diarrhoea.

Traditional vaccination methods use either a weakened or killed version of the disease- causing organism or a component of the organism, such as inactivated toxins or proteins. These component vaccines can either be purified from the organism itself or genetically engineered. The injection or oral administration of these non-disease-causing mimics mobilizes the immune system to protect the host form the disease.

DNA vaccination differs from traditional vaccines in that just the DNA coding for a specific component of a disease-causing organism is injected into the body. The DNA can be administered either in a saline solution injected through a hypodermic needle or on DNA-coated gold beads propelled into the body using gene guns. The actual production of the immaunizing protein takes place in a vaccinated host. This eliminates any risk of infection associated with some live and attenuated virus vaccines.

The report lists a number of other advantages DNA vaccines have over classic vaccine methods:

1. DNA vaccination provides long-lived immune responses, unlike many component vaccines that require multiple inoculations to maintain immunity.
2. Vaccines for multiple diseases can all be given in a single inoculation. Currently, in the United States, the full course of childhood immunizations require 18 visits to the doctor or clinic.
3. All DNA vaccines can be produced using similar techniques. The ability to use generic production methods greatly simplifies the vaccine development and production process.
4. They are extremely stable. Unlike many conventional vaccines that must be held at a constant temperature, DNA vaccines can be stored under a vast array of conditions either dried or in a solution. This eliminates the need for the "cold chain" – the series of refrigerators required to maintain a vaccine during distribution. This will greatly improve the

ability to deliver vaccines to remote areas in developing countries.

5. Candidate vaccines can be recovered from diseased tissue. Microbial DNA can be isolated from the tissue of an infected animal, purified, amplified and screened for vaccine candidates.

DNA vaccination may have its own limitations. The most obvious is that it is limited to developing immune responses against only the protein components of pathogens. The question of which vector to use also remains controversial. Moreover, some microbes have an outer shell made of polymerized sugars, known as polysaccharides. DNA vaccines cannot substitute for the more traditional polysaccharide-based vaccines, such as the pneumococcal vaccine for bacterial pneumonia.

Simplified Methodology of DNA Vaccination

This approach to immunization involves the direct introduction of a plasmid DNA encoding an antigenic protein gene which is then expressed within cells of the organism (3-6). The antigenic protein geneis isolated at first (Fig. 2.1). The introduction of the DNA can be accomplished by simple intramuscular or intradermal injections using needles, as well as by propelling DNA coated gold particles of various tissues (6), preferentially the dermis. Although very few cells can be transfected using these methods, the amount of protein produced as well as other parameters of the method (not all of which are understood) lead to surprisingly 112 immune respones (7), in the absence of any further adjuvant apart perhaps from the DNA itself (Fig. 2.2).

The responses include not only antibody induction and T-cell activation with cytokine secretion, but also the production of cytotoxic T lymphocytes (CTL). Most importantly of all, it has been shown in several instances that DNA-medicated immunization to a single antigen will provide protection against infection by a pathogen (1,7). Although DNA vaccines share the same limitations as a recombinant protein vaccines (*i.e.* the antigen conferring protection must in principle be known), this does not seem to be incompatible with achieving a fully protective immune response to at least some pathogens. Moreover, if combinations of antigens are required, then simple mixture of plasmids could conceivably be used.

FIGURE 2.1: Isolation of a Gene from Specific Antigenic Protein

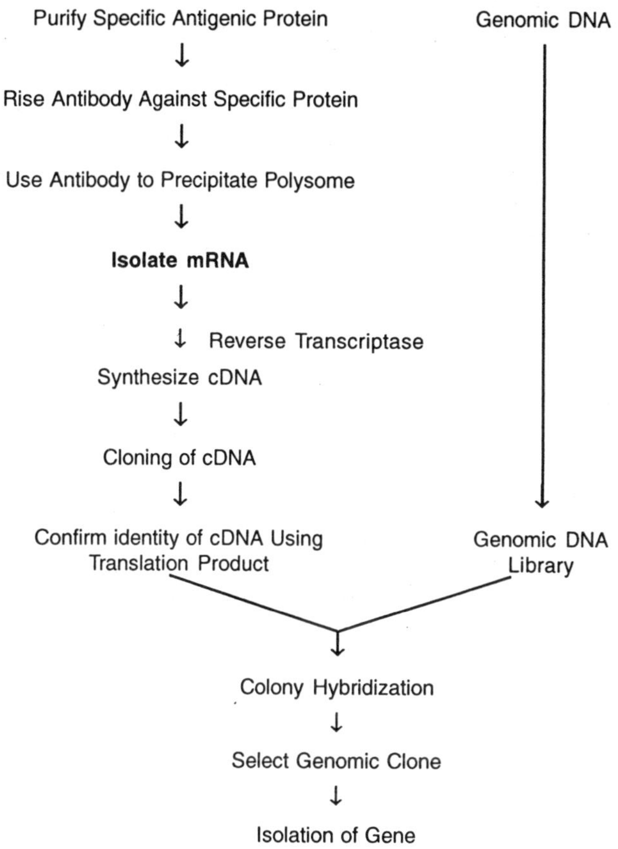

Plasmid DNA as Vector, Gene and Adjuvant Relation to DNA Vaccination

In addition to providing the coding sequences for antigenic protein, the plasmid also serves as the physical vector carrying the genes. More remarkable however is the possibility that DNA also serves as an adjuvant in the process of DNA-mediated

FIGURE 2.2: Flowchart of DNA Vaccination

Antigenic protein gene (DNA)

↓

Encoding the antigenic protein gene with a plasmid DNA

↓

DNA can be accomplished by simple intramascular or intraderminal injections using needles, as well as by propelling DNA-coated gold particles various tissues preferentially the dermis

↓

After injection, amount of protein produced as well as other parameters of the method (not all of which are understood) lead to surprisingly H2 immune responses. The responses include not only antibody induction and T-cell activation with cytokine secretion, but also the production of cytotoxic T-lymphocytes (CTL).

immunization. For decades, polynucleotides and even high molecular weight genomic DNA has served as non-specific stimulators of the immune system. Recent data has identified sequences in bacterial DNA that appear to specifically serve as a mitogen for B cells (15). In a more general way however, the large amount of DNA that accompanies an intramuscular injection but which does not function to express protein could be taken up by macrophage cells which would likely be stimulated to secrete interleukin-12. This cytokine could then impinge on natural killer cells to release interferon-γ which in turn would favour development of T-helper cells along the pathway to a TRI phenotype with further secretion of IL-2 and interferon-g. Such a cytokine environment would H2ly favour antigen processing by stimulating biochemical catabolism of the antigenic proteins encoded by the plasmid DNA.

Thus, a very attractive scenario can be envisioned for DNA immunization whereby favourable conditions are provided for antigen presentation by involving dendritic cells on one hand, and providing an cytokine environment which could further augment the efficiency of antigen processing and epitope presentation. Clearly the small amounts of protein that are made from introduced plasmids require the most efficient mechanisms to stimulate the impressive immune responses that have been observed. In some ways, the most surprising feature of this explanation is that one appears to have arrived at a remarkably efficient set of conditions for immunization in a totally serendipitous way.

Hepatitis B Surface Antigen and DNA Vaccination

The envelope protein of hepatitis B virus (HBV) can be expressed as three forms, each of which contains the same C-terminal 226 amino acids which carry the surface antigen determinants (HbsAg). The major form of the HbsAg-carrying protein (the S protein, or SHBs), contains all the topological information needed for panicle assembly (8). Such particles will form and are secreted when the gene for this protein is expressed in a variety of eukaryotic cell types. The surface antigen epitopes are conformational since they can only be induced by correctly formed particles. Further N-terminal extensions to the S protein are encoding by the preS region of the envelope gene, and additions of the preS2 sequence give rise to the middle or MHBs protein, while the entire pre region (preS2 + preS1) produces the large or LHBs polypeptide (2). The preS-containing forms are not used as precursor proteins, but rather are included as minor components in the secreted particles (MHBs) or the viral particles (MHBs and LHBs). The presence of these sequences in the particles provide additional B-and T-cell epitopes.

Most researchers have used plasmids containing the various envelope gene sequences under the control of the cytomegalovirus promote to express particles exclusively composed of the SHBs or of mixtures of SHBs and MHBs, or all three polypeptides (5,9). The plasmids were introduced into mice by intramuscular injection using an optimized protocol (10). The results of a serological analysis of the antibodies which were induced resulted in the conclusion that the envelope protein which was synthesized after DNA injection was in fact assembled into particles (9). The immune response also had many characteristics in common with the response to the HbsAg during natural infection by the virus. This type of conclusion is important since the protein is being synthesized by cells types (muscles fibrers and others) which are not the normal site of infection by the virus. This could in some cases interfere with correct processing and/or assembly of a protein from a pathogen whose gene is introduced into the vertebrate cells in this way.

CTL Responses and DNA Vaccination

The HBV envelope is able to induce class-I restricted CTL responses as an exogenous molecule (11). This may be related to the particulate state of the protein, since this property is thought to be important for such processing (12). Since DNA immunization has routinely been shown capable of inducing CTL activity in addition to humoral responses to the endoded proteins (2,7), it is possible that DNA based immunization using the HBsAg coding sequences will provide for CTL induction due to endogenous synthesis of the protein as well as a further CTL response coming from the exogenous protein.

It is not possible to explicitly determine whether exogenous HbsAg accounts for a large proportion of the CTL priming after DNA-based immunization. However, the fact that a H2 induction of cytotoxic activity was observed experimentally (13) suggests that whatever the process involved, the HbsAg protein could be an excellent carrier for other sequences for which a CTL response is being sought. DNA mediated immunization is so effective because the synthesized proteins access specialized antigen-presenting cells (APC) in a very efficient manner (14). These cells could be interstitial dendritic cells, which are the most efficient APC known and are found in many non-lymphoid tissues.

HbsAg Particles as Carriers of Heterologous Epitopes

Like many other self-assembling protein structures, HbsAg particles are candidates for carrying heterologous epitopes from other pathogens for the purpose of enhancing the immune response to those epitopes. Specifically, the epitope amino acid sequence is incorporated within the coding sequence of the carrier protein. This might be advantageous if the immune response to such epitopes would provide protection against infection and/or development of disease (16). The carrier particles probably serve at least two functions. They render the heterologous epitope multivalent since it is potentially part of each polypeptide of the carrier protein. The particles will themselves provide class II epitopes to provide T-help functions, and a characteristic of a good carrier will be one that provides efficient helper functions. The desirability of using a carrier for heterologous epitopes (which could even be rather large fragments of the heterologous antigen) arises if the antigenic protein under consideration is poorly immunogenic for reasons that can be related to the structure of the protein.

There are many uncertainties that arise from the considerations mentioned above, due to the many potential combinations of epitopes and carriers. It becomes quite clear that a simple methodology to test these various combinations will greatly benefit this approach. One illustration of this the fact that the large body of experimental data concerning the hepatitis B capsid protein as a carrier of heterologous epitopes surely arises from the fact that this protein can be expressed in *Escherichia coli* (17) and *Samonella typhimurium* (8). In contrast, chimeric HbsAg proteins require expression in mammalian cell cultures (16, 19), which is far more complicated, costly and time-consuming. It is therefore evident that the future use of DNA-based immunization will allow experimentation to benefit from the remarkable power of DNA manipulations and the great simplification that comes from direct plasmid DNA injection into experimental animals to assess modifications of carriers and their epitopes.

Our View for Some Important Points of DNA Vaccination

It is important that the method of DNA-mediated immunization become firmly entrenched as standard techniques in immunological practice. However, anecdotal reports indicate that the potential or the apparent experimental simplicity is not always fully realized in the hands of many investigators. Although the lack of a flood of papers using the method may indicate that it is simply still early days, it seems desirable to provide a step-by-step program of self-help for those who are endeavouring to overcome the pain of failed experiments (or failed collaborations). The some step program that we propose can be implemented as follows:

1. It is needed to fearlessly consider the nature of the sequences to be expressed if they are not viral genes or otherwise normal expressed in a mammalian cell. It must be noted that the sequences have any unusual codons or not and are there introns, and will they be correctly handled by the splicing machinery of the mammalian tissue?
2. There is an exercise wisdom in the choice of expression vector. The CMV and RSV promoters are the most likely to work (the plasmids pcDNA3 containing the CMV promoter and pRc/

RSV from Invitrogen are good ones to start with). However, if over expression of the protein is toxic then may be a weaker promoter (for examples SV40) would be better (20).

3. If the coding sequences inserted into the expression vector have been made by PCR, it needs to verify them by DNA sequencing.
4. If the vector contains a promoter sequence for a prokaryotic RNA polymerase (T7 or SP6 polymerase for example), it needs to consider preparing mRNA *in vitro* and carrying out reticulocyte cell-free translation to verify the fact that the protein can be synthesized by the mammalian translational machinery.
5. It is also necessary to carry out transient transfect of mammalian cells (such as COS, 3T3, or muscle cell lines if you wish) in order to verify the ability of the vector to correctly direct protein production after entry into a cell. So, detection can be simply carried out by immunofluorescence or by Western blotting. Alternatively, if the protein is supposed to be secreted, then it is necessary to assay the supernatant of the transfected cell culture.
6. If the vector is functional, then the intramuscular injection technique must be use and needs to choose a muscle that facilitates injection and examination (10, 21). It is needed to inject Indian ink first co-verify that the injection is indeed within the muscle (21). It is also needed to inject a control β-galactosidase plasmid (for example, pCMVb from Clontech) and stain the muscle for enzyme activity (10).
7. Then it is also needed to continue to validate intramuscular injection technique with respect to its ability to achieve immunization against a control protein using an existing plasmid. The HbsAg-expressing plasmid (5) is available from various institute, and the HbsAg antibodies can easily be detected with commercial clinical kits (from Abbott or Sanofi Diagnositics Pasteur for example) that can be used no matter what animal is being used for the DNA immunization. Since the antibody levels can be expressed in International Units, comparison can be made with previously published data.
8. Ultimately it is urgently needed to inject plasmid using the successful method that have worked out in 1 through 7.

Normally, if the plasmid functions and the protein is sufficiently antigenic, antibodies will being to be seen by 2 weeks and may well increase for up to 4 to 8 weeks (9).

9. If no antibody response to the antigen is seen after one month. It is necessary to keep the animals longer. Boosting with more plasmid DNA can be attempted although any defects in the DNA injection procedure must be promptly eliminated. It is possible that CTL activity might be present, although the lack of antibody response might be an important message about the ability of the system to work well.
10. PCR detection of the DNA is tempting to carry out, but presence of the DNA will not necessarily indicate that the detected DNA is actually in a form that is capable of being expressed (*e.g.* it may be extranuclear).
11. The most straightforward analysis at this point is to perform immunokfluorescence on transverse muscle sections to assess whether the protein was expressed by the muscle fibers *in vivo* (21). Alternatively, it might by possible to detect the protein in the circulation, or in a muscle tissue extract. However, these methods require very sensitive assay systems.

Although the above steps have been liberally adopted most of the researchers in their programs, there seems no reason to think that the various points highlighted above would not be beneficial to those wishing to enter the realm of DNA-mediated immunization.

New Oral DNA Vaccine for Trials

The International AIDS Vaccine Initiative (IAVI) will fund testing of a new kind of preventive vaccine, which has been developed at the Institute for Human Virology (IHV), started in 1996 by Robert Gallo at the University of Maryland. The new vaccine will be taken orally, and could possibly very low cost to produce.

Several aspects of this technology are particularly important:

1. There are many advantages to vaccines which work by delivering DNA which instructs cells to produce the specific proteins against which immunity is needed. But ordinarily DNA could not be taken orally because it would not reach the places it needs to go. The new technology uses a *Salmonella* bacterium which has been genetically modified so that it

does not cause disease and also genetically modified so that it includes selected parts of HIV.

The *Salmonella* bacterium "knows its way around the gut," and delivers the selected DNA directly to dendritic cells in the intestinal mucosa, which may be particularly effective for providing "mucosal immunity" to prevent HIV infection. This is important for blocking sexual transmission of the virus.

2. This bacterium has plenty of room to carry added DNA, allowing great flexibility for modifications. If the first vaccine does not work, different versions can easily be made by trying other parts of the virus. This vaccine can be customized for the different viral strains which cause epidemics in different pans of the world.
3. The six standard children's vaccines cost less than $1 to produce (for all six), but $15 or more per person to deliver in developing countries, because of the need for sterile injection, specially trained health workers, etc. An oral medication should be much less expensive to deliver.

This vaccine is well along in its development, but clinical trials are still more than a year away. The first trials will take place in Baltimore and in Uganda, where the Ministry of Health is an active participant.

Concluding Remark

From the study of model systems ill animals, there seems little doubt that DNA vaccines are a distinct possibility for the prevention of future infectious diseases in human populations. There are several obvious advantages of DNA vaccines. They are easier to manufacture than an inactivated pathogen, subcellular fraction or recombinant protein vaccines. Different plasmids encoding different antigens would be prepared in identical ways. The DNA is very stable and is resistant to extremes or temperature; thus storage, transport and distribution of DNA-based vaccines would be facilitated. In addition to these considerations for the commercial side of vaccine production and distribution, there are equally attractive advantages in the area of vaccine research and development. Seen from the point of view or molecular immunophysiology, it is now possible to modify the sequence of an antigenic protein, or to add heteriologous epitopes, by simple manipulations performed on the plasmid DNA. This can be followed by direct assessment of the changed immunogenicity of the protein after direct injection of the plasmid DNA. This simplifying methodology therefore promises to greatly enhance our ability to understand the structure-function relationships between the protein and the immune response to the antigen. In addition to enriching our knowledge of the molecular basis of the immune response, this type of understanding should also have a major impact on vaccine research. As new knowledge of the immune response is acquired, one could envision that modifications will be incorporated into proteins which could increase their antigenicity.

Acknowledgement

In the preparation of this chapter help has been taken from various source papers which has been duly acknowledged. We are also grateful to Dr. Robert G. Whalen from DNAVaccine.com for his kind help.

References

1. Ellis, R.W. (1993). *Hepatitis B vaccines in clinical practice*. New York, NY, Marcel Dekker.

2. Whalen, R.G., Davis, H.L. (1995). DNA-mediated immunization and the energetic immune response to hepatitis B surface antigen. *Clin. Immunol. Immunopathol.*, 75(1): 1-12.

3. Ulmer, J.B., Donnelly, J.J., Parker, S.E., Rhodes, G.H., Feigner, P.L., Dwarki, V.J., Gromkowski, S.H., Deck, R.R., DeWitt, C.M., Friedmana, A., Hawe, L.A., Leander, K.R., Martinez, D., Perry, H.C., Shiver, J.W., Montgomery, D.L., and Liu, M.A. (1993). Heterologous protection against influenza by injection of DNA encoding a viral protein. *Science*, 259: 1745-1749.

4. Wang, B., Ugen, K.E., Srikantin, V., Agadjanyan, M.G., Dang, K., Refaeli, Y., Sato, A.I., Boyer, J., William, W.V., Weiner, D.B. (1993). *Gene inoculation generates immune responses against human immunodeficiency virus type*. L. Proc, Natl. Acad, Sci., USA, 90; 4156-4160.

5. Davis, H.L., Michel, M.L., Whalen, R.G. (1993). DNA based immunization for hepatitis B induces continuous secretion of antigen and high levels of circulating antibody. *Human Molec. Genet.*, 2: 1847-1851.

6. Fynan, E.F., Webster, R.G., Fuller, D.H., Haynes, J.R., Santoro, J.C., Robinson, H.L. (1993). DNA vaccines, protective immunizations by parenteral, mucosal, and gene-gun incubations. *Proc. Natl. Acad. Sci.*, USA, 90(24): 11478-11482.

7. Davis, H.L., Whalen, R.G. (1995). DNA vaccination. In: Dickson, G. (ed) *Molecular and Cell Biology of Human Gene Therapeutics*. Chapman and Hall, London.

8. Gerlich, W.H., Bruss, V. (1993). Functions of hepatitis B virus proteins and molecular targets for protective immunity. In: Ellis, R.W. (ed) *Hepatitis B vaccines in clinical practice*. New York, NY, Marcel-Dekker, pp. 41-82.

9. Michel, M.L., Davis, H.L., Schleef, M., Mancini, M., Tiollais, P., Whalen, R.G. (1995). DNA mediated immunization to the hepatitis B surface antigen in mice: Aspects of the humoral response mimic hepatitis B viral infection in humans. *Proc. Natl. Acad. Sci.*, USA, 92: 5307-5311.

10. Davis, H.L., Demencix, B.A., Quantin, B., Coulombe, J., Whalen, R.G. (1993). Plasmid DNA is superior to virus vectors for direct gene transfer in adult muouse skeletal muscle. *Human Gene Ther.*, 4: 733-740.

11. Schirmbeck, R., Melber, K., Kuhrober, A., Janowiez, Z.A., Reimann, J. (1994). Immunization with soluble hepatitis B virus surface protein elicits murine H-2 class I-restricted CD8+cytotoxic T lymphocyte responses *in vivo*. *J. Immunol.*, 152(3): 1110-1119.

12. Kovacsovics-Bankowski, M., Rock, K.L. (1995). A phagosome-to-cytosol pathway for exogenous antigens presented on MHC class I molecules. *Science*, 267: 243-246.

13. Davis, H.L., Schirmbeck, R., Reimann, J., Whalen, R.G. (1995). DNA-mediated immunization in mice induces a potent MHC class I-restricted cytotoxic T lymphocyte response to the hepatitis B envelope protein. *Hum. Gene Ther.*, 6: 1447-1456.

14. Whalen, R.G., Leclerc, C., Deriaud, E., Schirmbeck, R., Reimann, J., Davis H.L. (1995). Activation and entrainment of the immune response after DNA-mediated immunization to the hepatitis B surface antigen. New York Academy of Sciences. 2(10): 38-96.

15. Holt, J.T. (1995). A 'senseless' immune response to DNA. *Nature Medicine*, 1(5): 407-408.

16. Michel, M.L., Mancini, M., Sobczak, E., Favier, V., Guetard, D., Bahraoui, E.M., Tiollais, P. (1988). Induction of anti-human immunodeficiency virus (HIV) neutralizing antibodies in rabbits immunized with recombinant HIV-hepatitis B surface antigen particles. *Proc. Natl. Acad. Science*, USA, 85: 7957-7961.

17. Borisova, G., Arya, B., Dislers, A., Borschukova, O., Tsibinogin, V., Skrastina, D., Eldnrov, M.A., Pumpens, P., Skryabin, K.G., Grens, E. (1993). Hybrid hepatitis B virus nucleocapsid bearing an immunodominant region from hepatitis B virus surface antigen. *J. Virol.*, 67(6): 3696-3701.

18. Schodel, F., Wirtz, R., Peterson, D., Hughes, J., Warren, R., Sadoff, J., Milich, D. (1994). Immunity to malaria elicited by hybrid hepatitis B virus core particles carrying circumsporozoite protein epitopes. *J. Exp. Med.*, 180(3): 1037-1046.

19. Michel, M.L., Pontisso, P., Sobczak, E., Malpiece, Y., Streeck, R.E., Tiollais, P. (1984). Synthesis in animal cells of hepatitis B surface antigen particles carrying a receptor for polymerized human serum albumin. *Proc. Natl. Acad. Sci.*, USA, 81: 7708-7712.

20. Xiang, Z.Q., Spitalnik, S., Tran, M., Wunner, W.H., Cheng, J., Ertl, H.C. (1994). Vaccination with a plasmid vector carrying the rabies virus glycoprotein gene induces protection immunity against rabies virus. *Virology*, 199(1): 132-140.

21. Davis, H.L., Whalen, R.G. (1993). Direct gene transfer into skeletal muscle *in vivo* factors affecting efficiency of transfer and stability of expression. *Hum. Gene Ther.*, 4(2): 151-159.

CHAPTER 3

PLASMID DNA PREPARATION An Approach Towards New DNA Vaccine Development

Introduction

Plasmid DNA (deoxyribonucleic acid) constitutes a new approach to vaccine development. DNA vaccines called Plasmid DNA vaccines, are the today's trend. So, this chapter review topics like plasmid DNA as vector, gene and adjuvant for new DNA vaccine development, regulations of plasmid DNA for DNA vaccine development, important aspects for plasmid DNA preparation what should be and should not be for plasmid DNA modifications, preparation of plasmid DNA by anion exchange chromatography for intramuscular injection, pre-clinical safety evaluation, clinical investigations and novel vaccine strategies using fowlpox viruses and plasmid DNA.

The use of purified preparations of plasmid DNA (deoxyribonucleic acid) constitutes a new approach to vaccine development. Plasmid DNA in DNA vaccines may find application as: preventive vaccines for viral, bacterial, or parasitic diseases; immunizing agents for the preparation of hyperimmune globulin products; therapeutic vaccines for infectious diseases; or for other indications such as cancer (1,6).

DNA vaccines called Plasmid DNA vaccines, are defined as purified preparations of plasmid DNA designed to contain a gene or genes for the intended vaccine antigen as well as genes incorporated into the construct to allow for production in a suitable host system. Plasmid DNA vaccines currently under development are constructs derived from bacterial plasmids that contain one or more genes from an infectious agent. These plasmids possess DNA sequences necessary for selection and replication in bacteria; eukaryotic promoters and enhancers; and transcription termination/ polyadenylation addition sequences for gene expression. However, because the current state of scientific knowledge with respect to the use of plasmid DNAs as preventive vaccines is limited. Plasmid DNA vaccines which are intended for use as preventive vaccines and therapeutic vaccines for infectious diseases.

Plasmid DNA as Vector, Gene and Adjuvant for New DNA Vaccine Development

In addition to providing the coding sequences for the antigenic protein, the plasmid also serves as the physical vector carrying the genes. More remarkable however is the possibility that DNA also serves as an adjuvant in the process of DNA-mediated immunization. For decades, polynucleotides and even high molecular weight genomic DNA has served as non-specific stimulators of the immune system. Recent data has identified sequences in bacterial DNA that appear to specifically serve as a mitogen for B cell (2). In a more general way however, the large amount of DNA that accompanies an intramuscular injection but which does not function to express protein could be taken up by macrophage cells which would likely be stimulated to secrete interleukin-12. This cytokine could then impinge on natural killer cells to release interferon-g which in turn would favour development of T-helper cells along the pathway to a Th1 phenotype with further secretion of IL-2 and interferon-g. Such a cytokine enviornment would H2ly favour antigen processing by stimulating biochemical catabolism of the antigenic proteins encoded by the plasmid DNA.

Thus, a very attractive scenario can be envisioned for DNA immunization whereby favourable conditions are provided for antigen presentation by involving dendritic cells on one hand, and providing an cytokine environment which could further augment the efficiency of antigen processing and epitope presentation. Clearly the small amounts of protein that are made from introduced plasmids require the most efficient mechanisms to stimulate the impressive immune responses that have been observed. In some ways, the most surprising feature of this explanation is that one appears to have arrived at a remarkably efficient set of conditions for immunization in a totally serendipitous way (Fig. 3.1).

Regulations of Plasmid DNA for DNA Vaccine Development

Development concerns associated with the use or plasmid DNA vaccines are similar to those for other biological products. Of concern is the source of the DNA incorporated into the vector, including eukaryotic promoters and enhancer; termination/polyadenylation

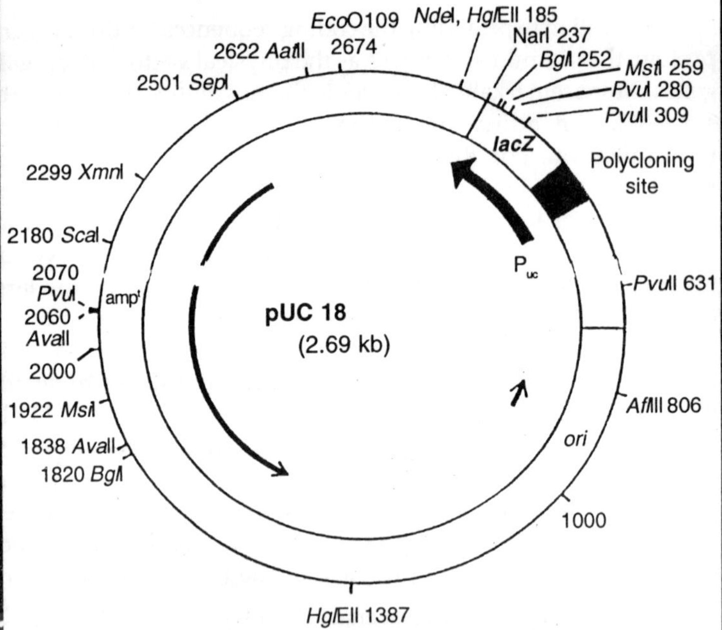

FIGURE 3.1: Plasmid DNA as Vector for DNA Vaccine

addition sites, antibiotic resistance markers; and other selection markers. In order to limit the possibility for chromosomal integration, homology of plasmid DNA sequence to know sequences in the human genome should be examined and described, and strong homology avoided if possible. Viral promoters and mammalian and viral termination and polyadenylation signals are frequently used, however, the results of expression and safety studies should dictate the choice of regulatory control sequences used in plasmid DNA constructs. Antibiotic resistance is commonly employed as a selection marker. In considering the use of an antibiotic resistance marker, it is advising manufacturers against the use of pencillin or other beta-lactam antibiotics as these antibiotics can, in certain individuals, result in allergic reactions ranging in severity from skin rashes to immediate anaphylaxis. When an antibiotic resistance marker is required in a plasmid DNA vaccine construct, Scientist board advises the use of an antibiotic such as kanamycin or neomycin. These aminoglycoside antibiotics are not extensively used the treatment of clinical infections due to their low activity spectrum, prevalence of kanamycin-resistant bacteria, and their problematic therapeutic index with toxicities including irreversible to toxicity and nephrotoxicity. Specifications for the level of antibiotic present in the final container should be established and should consider the minimum level of antibiotic that will give an unintentional clinical effect. The use of alternative antibiotic resistance markers or the use of suppressor tRNA genes in a plasmid construct intended as plasmid DNA vaccine.

Some Important Aspects for Plasmid DNA Preparation

Plasmid Vaccine Manufacture and Characterisation

When preparing a new plasmid DNA vaccine, the following specific product information should be noticed. The application should describe in detail the plasmid DNA vaccine vector construction, including the source and diagrams of all plasmids used, and all intermediate recombinanat DNA cloning procedures. Prior to licensure, the DNA sequence of the plasmid DNA should be provided for each vaccine construct by direct sequencing of the plasmid present in the Master Cell Bank. Preliminary clinical investigations may proceed with plasmid DNA products characterized using a combination of direct sequence and restriction enzyme mapping and polymerase chain reaction (PCR) may be employed at intermediate steps.

Specifications for the Bulk Plasmid Product

If bulk and final product are the same (*i.e.*, if production runs yield one lot and no further steps in formulation are performed), then testing as described below may be redundant and unnecessary. Bulk plasmid products should be tested for the properties described below. Standard assay(s) of adequate specificity and sensitivity can be used.

The DNA content in the bulk plasmid DNA vaccine and the presence of other cell-derived contaminants such as RNA (ribonucleic acid) and proteins should be evaluated. A test for homogeneity of size and determination of plasmid structure (*i.e.*, supercoiled vs. linear and relaxed circular DNA or concatamers should be performed). Agarose gel electrphoresis may be a useful technique to collect this information. A test for contaminating RNA or host DNA should also be included in the analysis. Blot hybridization techniques (Southern and Northern) in combination with gel electrophoresis will add to the sensitivity of the procedures. Appropriate tests to detect contaminating proteins also should be performed. The use of silver stained gels will provide a high degree of sensitivity to detect contaminating proteins and would be preferred over Coomassie Blue stained gels. In addition, immunologic techniques, such as enzyme-linked immunosorbent assay (ELISA) or Western blot, may be useful to detect contaminating host proteins.

The identity of the DNA plasmid vaccine may be determined by restriction enzyme digestion with multiple enzymes. A test for sterility to detect aerobic and anaerobic bacteria should be performed. Specific preclinical tests may be appropriate for products having specific safety concerns such as those DNA plasmid vaccines incorporating co-stimulatory cytokine genes or formulated with novel lipid or adjuvant components.

Whenever possible, potency assay should measure the level of production and immunogenicity of the gene product expressed by the plasmid vaccine.

Final Release Testing

During early product development and clinical investigation, specifications and criteria for lot release should be defined. Plasmid DNA vaccine products intended for phase 1 clinical studies should be tested for potency, general safety, sterility, purity, quantity, and identity. A test for potency may be an *in-vitro* or *in-vivo* test to evaluate the specific ability of the vaccine to effect a given response, such as an immune response in mice or the production of the pertinent antigen in a transfected cell line. A test for sterility should be performed. Other tests for quality of the final product should include an evaluation for residual moisture (required for licensed products) if the product is lyophilized, and a test for the presence of pyrogenic substances. Each lot of vaccine should be tested to establish the identity of the material in the final container. In addition to final product lot release, in-process testing should also be performed to ensure manufacturing consistency and product safety. Acceptance criteria and acceptable limits should be established and the results reported for each lot of vaccine to be used for clinical studies. For plasmid DNA vaccine products in their final container form, adventitious agent testing may be limted to sterility tests.

RNA, protein, and bacterial genomic DNA are possible contaminants that may be introduced during product manufacture, and the presence of these possible contaminants should be monitored in the product. Plasmid-derived DNA species such as linear and relaxed circular DNA may be less effective in expressing the inserted antigen gene. There should be a specification for the minimum amount of supercoiled DNA present. This parameter should be a major criterion measured during stability studies.

What should be and should not be for Plasmid DNA Modifications

Plasmid DNA Preventive Vaccine Vector Structure

Changes in a plasmid DNA vector, exclusive of the antigen gene intended for expression, may generally result in the plsamid vaccine being considered a new product. Alteration of a single base-pair in a control region of the DNA plasmid may alter its safety properties, in which case a full evaluation of safety in preclinical studies may be needed. Other alterations may not affect the safety profile of the plasmid DNA vaccine vector may be considered for abbreviated safety testing.

A change in the inserted gene with no change in the plasmid DNA vaccine vector may kin some cases be considered as a modification requiring only abbreviated testing. For example, if the same plasmid vector is used to express a series of related proteins, then the safety issues for each DNA plasmid vaccine are only those presented by the insert and its expressed product.

In some cases, preclinical testing such as tissue localization, assessment of germ line alteration, and animal pharmacology / toxicology studies may not need to be repeated. Instead, relevant safety studies could focus on safety related to expression of the inserted gene or genes. Possible adverse effects might include expression of the antigen gene in inappropriate tissue sites, over-expression, or unexpected immune responses, such as inappropriate modulation of the immune response resulting in immunopathology.

DNA Sequence Information

Initial phase 1 clinical investigations may be initiated with a complete restriction enzyme analysis of the plasmid vector and the DNA sequence of the inserted gene. In the case of multiple related plasmids, adequate characterisation may include sequencing of the inserted gene and enough sequence of flanking regions and control regions to characterize the insertion and verify integrity of flanking regions.

Lipids, Microsphere Encapsulation, Cytokines

The use of novel components and delivery systems, such as the use of novel cationic lipid preparations to enhance uptake and expression of a plasmid DNA vaccine administered by intranasal immunization, may necessitate specific preclinical evaluation to ensure safety. The use of specialized delivery systems such as the encapsulation of the plasmid DNA vaccine in poly (UL-lactide-coglycolide) (PLG) microspheres may also necessitate preclinical evaluation. Similar considerations apply if other components, such as cytokine genes, are added to plasmid DNA vaccine vectors.

Preparation of Plasmid DNA by Anion Exchange Chromatography for Intramuscular Injection

Following steps are followed for Intramuscular Injection (5)

1. DNA is eluted from Qiagen column (the procedure is carried out following precisely the Quaigen protocol AND using the buffers provide by Quaigen). After isopropanol precipitation, the ethanol wash, and vacuum drying, the DNA is taken up in standard IX TE (Sigma). This is

conveniently left overnight to redissolve, although it will dissolve more rapidly if needed.

DNA from a CsCL gradient is extensively dialyzed versus IX TE. (N.B. Qiagen-prepared DNA is essentially as good as DNA prepared by two rounds of CsCl gradients).

2. Add NaCl to the DNA-TE solution to a final concentration of 0.1 M.
3. Then add 2 volumes of absolute ethanol. Precipitate at –20 degrees Centrigrade for 30 minutes and recover pellet by centrifugation.
4. Wash once with 70 per cent ethanol in water (no EDTA) and recover by centrifugation. If the DNA is to be sent to someone, send it in as the EtOH precipitate under the 70 per cent EtOH solution.
5. Dry the pellet, and resuspend it in IX sterile PBS (Sigma). From the size of the Qiagen column used, one can estimate the amount to DNA to be recovered and add the PBS to obtain a solution of about 1.5 to 2.0 mg/ml. At this point, it is best to leave DNA –PBS overnight at 4°C to dissolve. It is also very helpful to have the precipitate in a round bottom 15 ml to increase contact between dried DNA and PBS. If necessary, DNA-PBS can be warmed at 37 degrees Centigrate to speed up dissolution.
6. Read OD 260 and 280; the 260/280 ratio should be > 1.7 for a good DNA prep. Dilute the DNA to 1 mg/ml (or appropriate concentration). If necessary, store at –20 degrees Centigrade or colder.
7. DNA is now ready for injection.

The plasmids were introduced into mice by intramuscular injection using an optimized protocol (1). The results of a serological analysis of the antibodies which were induced resulted in the conclusion that the envelope protein which was synthesized after DNA injection was in fact assembled into particles (3).

We have used plasmids containing the various envelope gene sequences under the control of the cytomegalovirus promoter to express particles exclusively composed of the SHBs or of mixtures of SHBs and MHBs, or all three polypeptides (4, 3).

Pre-clinical Safety Evaluation

General Considerations

The preclinical evaluation of plasmid DNA vaccines is an important aspect of their development as candidate vaccine products. In designing preclinical studies, the primary consideration should be the intended clinical use, since the primary goal of preclinical studies is to obtain enough relevant data to allow initiation of a phase I clinical study. Both *in-vivo* and *in-vitro* studies may be employed to assess whether the product may be used safely in clinical studies. The type, duration, and scope of animal studies and other tests will vary with the duration and nature of the proposed clinical investigations. For example, a preventive vaccine intended for one-time administration will have supporting data different from a therapeutic vaccine that may be administered repeatedly. The use of non-traditional animal models of disease or challenge studies may also be useful for certain indications. Relevant animal models may also include the use of aged animals for the evaluation of vaccines proposed for use in elderly populations.

Immunogenicity Evaluation

During the preclinical development of these new vaccines, researchers should develop adequate assays for the assessment of the immunological potency of the vaccine.These results will be useful in choosing a proposed dose for clinical studies. The preclinical studies should be designed to assess the immune response, including seroconversion rares, geometric mean rates, geometric mean antibody titers and, if possible, cell-medicated immune responses in vaccinated animals. These studies should also be designed to collect information regarding the duration of antigen expression and whether long-term expression will result in tolerance or autoimmunity. Where appropriate and when possible, animal challenge/protection studies with the corresponding infectious agent are encouraged early in development to demonstrate the rationale for the use of the investigational vaccine. For those DNA plasmid vaccine constructs that co-express cytokine genes, specific preclinical studies should be considered to assess whether modulation of the cellular or humoral components of the immune system might result in unintended adverse consequences, such as generalized immunosuppression, chronic inflammation, autoimmunity or other immunopathology. When plasmid DNA vaccines are used in vaccination strategies employing a corresponding sub-unit vaccine, such as in prime and boost study designs, specific preclinical information should be submitted to support the schedule and route of administration with each vaccine combination.

Local Reactogenicity and Systemic Toxicity Studies

Studies designed to assess systemic toxicity may be combined with the assessment of local site reactogenicity. The design of these studies should include dose-ranging and dose-escalation, considering the anticipated dose and schedule of administration in clinical studies. The assessments written into the preclinical study protocols should include toxicity to potential target organs, including the hematopoietic and immune systems. Preclinical studies should also include clinical pathology, gross evaluations, and histopathology of tissues.

Local site reactogenicity studies should include detailed clinical and histological evaluations of injection-site tissue obtained form biopsies or term necropsy samples. Studies should be designed to assess the distribution or tropism of the vaccine for specific tissues. These studies should define the duration of the vaccine immunogen expression and persistence of the vector in somatic cells containing the plasmid DNA in DNA vaccine. The preclinical studies should be designed to determine whether the plasmid DNA in vaccine has an immunotoxic effect, either by inducing tolerance to the antigen encoded by the vaccine or by inducing autoimmunity. These studies should also be designed to assess whether antibody responses are elicited to contaminating bacterial proteins in the vaccine.

Genetic Toxicity

Integration of the plasmid DNA in DNA vaccine into the genome of the vaccinated subjects is an important theoretical risk to consider in preclinical studies. The concern is that an integrated vaccine may result in insertional mutagenesis through the activation of oncogenes or inactivation of tumor suppressor genes. In addition, an integrated plasmid DNA in vaccine may result in chromosomal instability through the induction of chromosomal breaks or rearrangements. The performance of a preclinical study to assess integration should focus on the potential of the plasmid DNA with DNA vaccine to recombine with endogenous host DNA sequences.

Studies designed to address the potential for integration should use the most sensitive methods available. For example, PCR studies using primers derived from the vaccine can be used to examine tissue distribution and to distinguish between integrated versus non-integrated plasmids in genomic DNA preparations. Use of separative electrophoretic methods can assist in the preparation of genomic DNA samples free of contaminating plasmids for use in such a study as can the use of rare restriction sites engineered into plasmid construct.

Localization studies designed to determine the distribution of the DNA plasmid vaccine after administration should be performed. Whenever feasible, testing should include both the intended route of administration (*e.g.* subcutaneous, intramuscular, intradermal, intranasal), as well as a group of animals treated intravenously, as a "worst-case" scenario. The presence of the DNA plasmid vaccine in surrounding and distal tissues as well as the vaccination site should be evaluated using the most sensitive detection methods available. If aberrant or unexpected localization occurs, studies should be conducted to determine whether the presence of the DNA plasmid vaccine is associated with a pathologic response. The studies should also include evaluation of the persistence of both the gene and its product in the target and non-target organs. The effects of over expression of antigen from the DNA plasmid vaccine should also be considered. Aberrant expression of some proteins may lead to an inappropriate activation of the immune system, resulting the generation of acute or chronic inflammatory responses, autoimmune sequelae, and destruction of normal tissues. Where generation of an autoimmune response is potentially a risk in either a long enough period to allow development of these disorders to appear.

Reproductive Toxicity Studies

Plasmid DNA preventive vaccines should be evaluated for migration to gonadal tissue and possible germline alterations in both male and female animals. This may be assessed through the performance of PCR on gonad-derived DNA preparations from male and female animals vaccinated with a plasmid DNA with DNA vaccine. Additional studies may be needed if the product is expected to affect normal physiological processes related to fertility, maintenance of pregnancy, or fetal development and will depend on factors such as the age and health status of the proposed subject population and the intended use.

Tumorigenicity Studies

Tumorigenicity studies may be appropriate under certain conditions. A tumorigenicity study should be considered if the results of the preclinical studies to assess integration of the plasmid DNA vaccine provide clear evidence of integration activity or broad tissue distribution, or if the vaccine is intended for chronic use in non-life threatening clinical situations. This type of study may also be relevant if the plasmid DNA in DNA vaccine construct has extensive DNA sequence homology to the human genome or if the vector contains sequences of known oncogenic potential. Manufacturers should carefully evaluate whether to proceed with product development should their particular construct exhibit integration activity.

Clinical Investigations

The data needed to support phase 1 trials should focus on safety, though some demonstration of immunogenicity is expected. Additional data from more detailed testing and results of process validation will be needed at later stages in product development as well as additional evidence of potency and efficacy. Sometimes product formulation is changed as product development progresses. In this case, comparability of the different formulations should be demonstrated by quantitative assays including biological potency testing.

Novel Vaccine Strategies Using Fowlpox Viruses and Plasmid DNA

Studies have been made on avipox viruses encoding cytokine genes, both alone and in combination with naked DNA plasmids, as potential vaccine strategies. As these viruses abortively infact mammalian cell, yet still effectively present foreign genes to the immune system, they offer a safer but effective alternative to other live vectors. We have examined the effect of co-expressing the cytokines interleukin-6 (IL-6) or interferon-gamma (IFN gamma) or immune responses to fowlpox virus (FPW) expressing influenza hemagglutinin (HA) as a vaccine antigen. IL-6 agumented antibody responses while IFN gamma inhibited these responses without affecting the generation of cell-mediated immunity. The safety of these constructs was demonstrated in immunodeficient mice and no side effects were observed due to cytokine expression. Direct injection of DNA plasmids encoding foreign genes as a means of vaccination is a subject of great current interest. We have combined this approach with fowlpox vectors, both expressing common HA antigen, to examine the effects of priming with the former intramuscularly and boosting with the recombinant FPV. With this combination, both systemic and mucosal antibody responses, respectively, were greatly elevated after boosting at the relevant site. Levels of systemic antibody achieved using this strategy approximated those in convalescent serum. In summary, FPV vectors encoding cytokines represent a safe and effective vaccine strategy which may be used to selectively manipulate the immune response. Greatly enhanced immune responses can be generated when this approach is used in combination with naked DNA immunisation. These findings have implications for the development of improved vaccination strategies.

Conclusion

This document is intended to provide manufacturers with information on concerns that are associated with the new technology of plasmid DNA preventive vaccines and to provide early guidance to the regulated industry. The goal is to create a regulatory environment that will encourage innovation and at the same time ensure that products are both safe and effective.

Acknowledgement

In the preparation of this chapter help has been taken from various source papers which has been duly acknowledged. We are also grateful to authorities of *DNAVaccine.com* for their kind help.

References

1. Davis, H.L., Demeneix, B.A., Quantin, B., Coulombe, J., Whalen, R.G. (1993). Plasmid DNA is superior to viral vectors for direct gene transfer in adult mouse skeletal muscle. *Human Gene Ther.*, 4: 733-740.

2. Holt, J.T. (1995). A 'senseless' immune response to DNA. *Nature Medicine*, 1(5): 407-408.

3. Michel, M.L., Davis, H.L., Schleef, M., Macini, M., Toillais, P., Whalen, R.G. (1995). DNA-mediated immunization to the

hepatitis B surface antigen in mice: Aspects of the humoral response mimic hepatitis B viral infection in humans. *Proc. Natl. Acad. Sci.,* USA, 92: 5307-5311.

4. Davis, H.L., Michel, M.L., Whalen, R.G. (1993). DNA based immunization for hepatitis B induces continuous secretion of antigen and high levels of circulating antibody. *Human Molec. Genet.,* 2: 1847-1851.
5. Nordston, K., Austin, S.J. (1989). Mechanism that contributes stable segregation of plasmids. *Annu. Rev. Genet.,* 23: 37-69.
6. Summers, D.K. (1996). *Plasmid Biology.* Blackwell Science, Oxford.

CHAPTER 4

Molecular (Protein and Non-Protein) Engineering for Designing of New Drugs

Introduction

Molecular (protein and non-protein) engineering is very necessary today, for designing of new drugs. One of the four methods is followed for drug designing, where designing by blocking enzyme activity, designing through blocking hormone receptor, designing through inhibition of nuclic acid synthesis and designing of peptide vaccine are considered. Some steps are followed for this engineering which includes characterization of the protein (or non-protein) within a ligand; its 3D structure study with NMR, X-ray diffraction, analysis and computer graphics study. The new drug is then characterised biochemically and then it is tested into a biological system.

A variety of molecules have evolved over a period of three billion years to yield the present day proteins and non-proteins which carry out complex function in the cells of all organisms. Molecular (protein and non-protein) engineering is the foremost among the many recent advances in biotechnology which reflect the exciting possibilities of proteins and nuclic acid conformation, modifications of the *de nove* design of a protein in a living system (6, 7).

Based on application as a drug, the new design is incorporated into protein or non- protein molecule. Newly engineered molecules have to be tested for their activity and then applied as drug into a targeted system (9,3,9). This chapter concludes with brief description about the steps of designing, process of designing and the newly engineered molecule in medicine industry.

Methods for New Drug Designing

Mainly one of the four methods are used for new drug designing.

Drug Designing by Blocking Enzyme Activity

Most of the drugs act by modifying of blocking the activity of an enzyme. So, in this method, the rational drug is designing for blocking the targeted enzyme. A drug like trimethorprim (TMP) is an important example which inhibits the activity of dihydrofolate reductase (dHFR) (4). Inhibitor of the enzyme of renin is also actively modelled. HIV proteinase inhibitor is also designed (8) Table 4.1.

Drug Designing Through Blocking Hormone Receptor

Drugs have also been produced for blocking hormone receptor molecules. That are responsible for diseases. Utilizing the strategy important two drugs *i.e.* propranolol (for treating heart disease and high blood pressure) and climatidine (antiulcer) were developed by J. Block, G. Elion and G. Hitchings for which they got Nobel Prize for physiology and medicine in the year 1988 (4) Table 4.1.

Drug Designing Through Inhibition of Nuclic Acid Synthesis

These drugs inhibit the nuclic acid (DNA or RNA) the pathogens or targeted cell. So, a detail study is needed for separating the pathways of nuclic acid synthesis between host and pathogen. Such type of drugs are 'pyramethamine' for malaria, 'trimethorpim' for bacterial infection and 'acyclovir' for herpes virus infection which inhibits the DNA synthesis of the pathogens. Some drugs (6-mercaptopurine) are going to be designed to inhibit the nuclic acid synthesis of cacerous cells (5,7) Table 4.1.

Designing of Peptide Vaccine

Recombinant DNA techniques have been used to synthesis of oligopeptides which would mimic with epitopies, thus invoking immune response. These short peptides can be designed for using as a vaccine in conjugation with carrier protein (8).

TABLE 4.1: Some Newly Engineered Protein and Non-Protein Molecule in Medicine Industry

Name of the Drug	*Application*	*Method Followed*
Inhibitor of renin	Lead to elevated blood pressure	By blocking enzyme activity
Trimethoprim	Treatment for urinary tract infection	By blocking enzyme activity
Propranolol	Treatment of heart disease, anginapectoris, high blood pressure	Through blocking hormone receptor
Climatidine	Antiulcer	Through blocking hormone receptor.
6-mercaptopurine	Cancer chemotherapy	Inhibit nuclic acid synthesis
Thiognanine	Cancer chemotherapy	Inhibit nuclic acid synthesis
Azathioprine	Rhematoid arthritis	Inhibit nuclic acid synthesis
Pyramethamine	Treatment of malaria	Inhibit nuclic acid synthesis
Trimethorpim	Treatment of bacterial infection	Inhibit nuclic acid synthesis
Acyclovir	Herpes virus infection	Inhibit nuclic acid synthesis
Azidothymidine (AZT)	For AIDS	Inhibit nuclic acid synthesis

Steps of Designing

According to Blundell (1989), (1), the basic out line of molecular (mainly protein) engineering involves characterized the protein with a ligand (*e.g.* enzyme-substrate, receptor-hormone etc.), 3D structure study through NMR (nuclear magnetic resonance) and x-ray diffraction, detailed study of 3D structure through computer graphics. With the available information, designing of the molecule (drug/vaccine) is to be done when the designed DNA sequence, suitable expressions systems, and the gene product are considered *i.e.* at last characterised biochemically (Fig. 4.1).

The knowledge about the site structure upto the level of atomic resolutions is needed, so that the accessible surface, which needs to be attacked, is known. A ligand will has to be designed that will fit the binding site, for this purpose the steric out line of the ligand should be complementary to the site so that this part (complementary

FIGURE 4.1: Steps of Molecular (Protein and Non-protein) Engineering for Designing of New Drugs

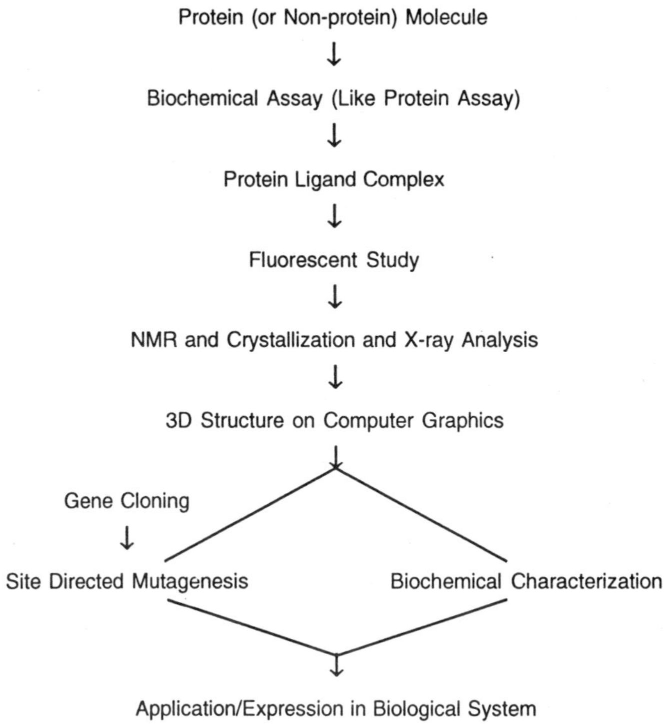

features) will have built in the ligand at appropriate position(s). This should result the maximum interactions between atoms of the ligand and the site. This process is successfully achieved with the help of computer aided methods. Once the ligand is designed for fitting the binding site, the ligand is to be modified to have pharamacological properties to maintain its affinity for the binding site (2). The whole process will require three dimensional (3D) constructions. Computer have provided methods which will allow automatic site director drug designing, is called computer aided molecular modelling (CMM).

Possible Engineered Drug for Future

Some molecule whose structures are known and cloned genes are available, so that they are used for protein and non-protein engineering. Those are mainly immunoglobulins, glucose isomerases, amylases, repressor proteins and restriction endonucleases.

Concluding Remark

New drug designing is cooperative endeavour between biochemists, crystallographers, computer scientist and molecular biologists. Exciting times are ahead for protein and non-protein molecules engineering for new drug development. Advances in technology and in understanding the principles of protein and nuclic acid structure and their design which will allow us to design, engineer and produce novel drugs with novel function. The impact of this protein and non-protein engineering on the near future of mankind will be at least a transistor or like small computer chips or probably more.

Acknowledgement

I am grateful to Dr. A.C. Banerjee, East India Pharmaceuticals Ltd.; Dr. T.K. Chatterjee, Deputy Directors, Zoological Survey of India and Dr. S.K. Chakraborty, Head, Dept. of Zoology, Vidyasagar University for their encouragement.

References

1. Blundell, T.L. (1989). Protein engineering and design. *Phil. Trans. Roy. Soc. Lond.*, B 324: 447-460.
2. Danziger, D.J. and Dean, P.M. (1989). Automated site directed drug design. *Phil. Trans. Roy. Soc. Lond.*, B236: 101-162.
3. DeGrado, W.F., Wasserman, Z.R. and Lear, J.D. (1989). Protein design, a minimalist approach. *Science*, 243: 622-628.
4. Gupta, P.K. (1994). Protein engineering, immunotoxins and drug designing. In: *Elements of Biotechnology*. Rastogi and Company, Meerut, (India), 437-457.
5. Horn, A.S. and De Ranter, C.J. (1984). *X-ray crystallography and drug action*. Clarendon Press.

6. Janny, B. (1988). Exploting the insights from protein structure. *Science*, 240: 722-723.

7. Knight, P. (1990). Non-protein engineering: Small drug design. *Biotechnology*, 8: 105-107.

8. Pattabhi, V. and Gautam, N. (1996). Protein engineering and design. In: *Concepts in Biotechnology*, Universities Press Ltd., Hyderabad, India, 89-113

9. Ring, D. (1989). Protein engineering: The sheep in wolf's clothing. *Nature*, 339: 658-659.

CHAPTER 5

BACTERIAL ADHESINS-BASED SURFACE PROTEIN

Today's Targets for New Vaccine Development

Introduction

Blocking the primary infection (mainly bacterial attachment to host cell receptors and colonization of the mucosal surface) may be the most effective strategy to prevent bacterial infections. Bacterial attachment involves through an interaction between a bacterial surface protein (adhesin) and the host cell receptor. Recent vaccine studies with adhesin have confirmed that antibodies elicited against an adhesin can impede colonization, block infection, and prevent disease. The chapter reviews the adhesin types in both from the gram positive and gram negative bacteria and the prophylactic vaccination with adhesins that can block bacterial infections.

The Principal aim of new vaccine development is to produce long-term protective immune responses against a pathogen. These responses include systemic humoral antibodies that neutralize in vasive organisms and cytotoxic T cells, which are required to clear certain infections, particularly chronic viral infections such as HIV (1). Helper T-cell and cytokine responses also influence humoral and cellular immune responses (2). For most bacteria and viruses, the first encounter with their host invloves attachment to a eukaryotic cell surface, which results the colonization of the host prior to disease. In such cases, induced antibody responses at the mucosal surface could prevent attachment and colonization. The ideal target for such antibodies surface proteins known as adhesins – mediate microbial attachment to host tissue (3). Studies with adhesin, the FimH protein from *Escherichia coli*, show that anti-adhesin antibodies can block microbial attachment and subsequent disease.

Furthermore, while specific induction of immune responses along the mucosal surface by mucosal immunization may have its advantages (4-7). The FimH studies demonstrate the immunoglobulin G (Ig) antibodies alone, which transudate into secretions after parenteral vaccination with the FimH adhesin, are sufficient to block colonization and infection. This chapter presents the role of Adhesins in microbial pathogenesis, Gram-Negative organisms and their Adhesins, Gram-Positive organisms and their Adhesins Bacterial adhesins for determinants of microbial colonization and pathogenicity, mucosal immune system for fundamental concepts to vaccine development and an approaches towards Adhesin-vaccines to block colonization.

Adhesins in Microbial Pathogenesis

To inititate infection, bacterial pathogens must first be able to colonize an appropriate target tissue of the host (8, 9). This tropism (ability to gain access to a niche within the body), in association with the ability of the bacterium to breach mucosal barriers and invade the host.

Colonization begins with the attachment of the bacterium to receptors expressed by cells forming the lining of the mocosa (Fig. 5.1). Certain species of bacteria are restricted in terms of the hosts and tissues they infect and the diseases they cause. In many cases, tropism for specific tissues has been corroborated in the laboratory by *in-vitro* binding assays with isolated epithelial cells collected from sites of infection or from infection-prone hosts.

Attachment is mediated by adhesin proteins; bacterial lectins are the most common type of adhesin among both gram-negative and gram-positive bacteria (3, 10-12). Adhesins, such as the FimH adhesin produced by most Enterobacteria ceae (including uropathogenic *E. coli*), are highly conserved proteins (13). Minor changes in the adhesin protein have been observed (2 per cent divergence) and correlate with decreased or increased affinity for binding to sugars (14), antibodies against a single FimH protein cross-react with > 90 per cent of *E. coil* strains expressing the FimH adhesin and block binding to bladder cells *in-vitro* (15, 16). However, antibodies against FimH from a single isolate protect against *in vivo* colonization by > 90 per cent of uropathogenic strains in a murine model for cystitis. This high degree of antigenic conservation is another reason why adhesins may serve as ideal vaccines.

Beside from mediating colonization of the host, bacterial attachment often results in the up-regulation or expression of many other virulence genes encoding various proteins that allow for invasion of the host (Figure 5.1) (17-23). The proteins can mediate tighter associations with epithelial cells, trigger epithelial cell-actin filament rearrangements, and induce changes in most-cell signaling the function. In some cases, the bacteria may also secrete a protein that inserts into mammalian cells and serves as a receptor for its own intimate adherence with the host (Figure 5.1) (24). Given that cross-talk between pathogenic bacteria and host cells after microbial attachment may trigger expression of virulence factors leading to local inflammation or evasive disease, vaccines that block bacterial attachment may have multiple advantages.

Many studies have demonstrated the utility of vaccines against bacterial surface components in blocking attachment *in-vitro* as well as *in-vivo* (25-28). However, as understanding of the mechanisms of attachment has evolved and characterization of specific adhesin molecules has been refined, new opportunities have emerged for the development or adhesin-based vaccines.

Gram-Negative Organisms and Their Adhesins

One of the best understood mechanisms of bacterial adherence in attachment mediated by cell surface structures called pili or fimbriae, a long, flexible structures that allow for contact between the bacteria and the host cell. Originally pili were thought to be homopolymeric structures composed of approximately 1,000 copies of a single structural subunit (fimbrin) packed in a helical array, however, for many pili, such as the highly characterized Type I and Pap pili expressed on *E. coli* and other *Enterobacteriaceae,* they are heteropolymeric structures with minor tip fibrillae proteins located at the distal end of the organelle (11). The specific interaction with receptor architectures on host cell surfaces is mediated by one of these tip proteins, called adhesins. For example FimH adhesin mediates attachment is occurred by type I pili (29, 30), while PapG mediates binding is occurred to the receptors on host cells by Pap pili (31, 32) (Table 5.1). The specificity of interaction may be involved in conferring tropism to the bladder and kidney tissues, respectively (33, 38). Pilus- associated adhesins have been identified in a number of other bacteria as well (Table 5.1).

Not all adhesins are associated with pili. *Bordetella pertussis* expresses at least two putative adhesins on its surface: filamentous hemagglutinin (FHA) and pertactin (34). FHA is thought to mediate attachment to sulfated sugars on cell-surface geycoconjugates, although it may also have other properties. Pertactin is thought to mediate binding by the Arg-Gly-Asp triplet binding sequence characteristic of integrin-binding proteins, although the role of this binding activity in the pathogenesis of *Bordetella* infections is unclear. Both FHA and pertactin are components in the recently approved a cellular pertussis vaccine.

In *Haemophilus influenzae,* two families of nonpilus adhesins have been identified: high-molecular weight adhesion proteins (HMW 1 and HMW 2) and immunogenic high molecular-weight surface-exposed proteins, the prototypic member of which has been designated Hia for *H. influenzae,* adhesin (35). Both families are expressed by nontypable *H. influenzae,* which colonized the respiratory tract and cause such diseases as otitis media, pneumonia, and bronchitis. The HMW proteins, which share homology with the *B. pertussis* FHA protein, medicine specific attachment of *H. influenzae* to different types of human epithelial cells *in vitro* and have been implicated in directing respiratory tract tropism for these organisms. The Hia protein, contrast, mediates tight association with human conjunctival cells and is present only in *H. influenzae* strains deficient in HMW 1/HMW 2 expression (36). Given the dichotomy among nontypable strains expressing either HM 1 or Hia-like adhesins and the serologic conservation at least among the HMW 1 and HMW 2 proteins, a vaccine based on a combination of such proteins may be protective against disease caused by most nontypable H. *influenzae.*

TABLE 5.1: Adhesins of Gram-negative Bacteria

Adhesion	*Strain*	*Ligand*	*Reference*
Pili family[1]			Hultgren (33)
PapG	*Escherichia coli*	Gala(1-4)Gal in globoseries of glycolipids	
SfaS	. *E. coli*	a-sialy1-2 3-b-galactose	
FimH	*E. coli*	Mannose-oligosaccharides	
HifE	*Hoemophilus Influenzae*	Sialylyganglioside-GM1	
PrsG	*E. coli*	Gala(1-4)Gal in globoseries of glycolipids	
MrkD	*Klebstella pneumoniae*	Type V collagen	
FHA	*Bordetella pertussis*	Sulfated sugars on cell-surface glycoconjugates	Brennan (34)
Pertactin	*B. pertussis*	Integrins	Brennan (34)
HMW1/HMW2	*H. influenzae*	Human epithelial cells	St. Geme (35)
Hia	*H. influenzae*	Human conjunctival cells	Barenkamp (36)
Le^b-binding Adhesin	*Helicobacter* pylori	Fucosylated Le^b histo-blood group Antigens	Ilver (37)

[1] Representative examples from the large family of pilus-associated adhesions; FHA: Filamentous hemagglutinin; HMW: High molecular weight; Hia: *H. influenzae* adhesin.

Another nonpilus adhesin has been identified and purified from *Helicohacter pylori*. The adhesin, called Le^b-binding adhesin, mediates bacterial adherence to fucosylated Lewis b (Le^b) histoblood group antigens, which are expressed along the mucosal surface of the gastric eipthelium (37). The Le^h-binding adhesin may be involved in conferring tropism for stomach epithelium and allowing pathogenic bacteria to establish an ecologic niche within the gastrointestinal tract. In association with other virulence determinants expressed by *H. pylori* in the stomach, the colonization process ultimately results in ulcer formation.

A unique mechanisms have been identified by which certain strains of enteropathogenic *E. coli* that cause severe diarrhoea target cells for attachment: Enteropathogenic *E. coli* express and insert their own receptor (Hp90) into mammalian cell surfaces, thereby allowing the bacteria to attach and establish intimate contact with the epithelial cells (24) (Figure 5.1). Although a bacterially encoded receptor for a cognate adhesin protein (intimin), Hp90 is expressed and secreted by enteropathogenic *E. coli* before colonization; therefore, it may also serve as a target for vaccine development.

FIGURE 5.1: Four Mechanisms of Bacterial Adherence where Anti-adhesin Vaccines could Potentially Block Colonization and Infection

Adherence where anti-adhesin vaccines could Potentially Block Colonization and Infection

1. Pili or fibrillae protruding from the bacterial surface. These proteinaceous appendages bind to host cell surface molecules, usually carbohydrates, by adhesin proteins located at the distal tip of the pilus-fibrillar organelle. Antibodies targeting the adhesin protein block the bacterial/host interaction.
2. A similar process of bacterial/epithelial cell interactions mediated by afimbrial adhesin proteins. In this case, antibodies directed against the bacterial surface proteins should also block attachment and colonization by impeding the ability of the bacteria to associate with mucosal tissues.
3. Some bacteria establish intimate association with eukaryotic cells by intimin proteins, resulting in cytoskeletal rearrangements, host cell signalling, possible internalization of the bacteria, and in many cases systemic disease. Blocking the intimate association/adherence may also be another strategy to prevent bacterial infections.
4. A novel mechanism whereby bacteria secrete their own receptor protein, which is internalized by the target host cell, phosphorylated, and embedded in the eukaryotic cell as a new receptor for tight binding by the bacterium. Theoretically, blocking the secreted receptor (Hp90) before it is internalized by the host cell could provide another mechanism to block bacterial adherence and infection.

Gram-Positive Organisms and their Adhesins

Some of the most well-characterized colonization factors in gram-positive bacteria –the polypetides of the antigen I/II family– bind to salivary glycoproteins in a lectinlike interaction (11) and promote adhesin to the tooth surface (Table 5.2). These proteins include the original AgI/II from *Streptococcus mutans,* also known as SpaP, PI, or Pac, and the *Streptococcus sobrinus* SpaA and Pag proteins (39). *Streptococcus gordonii* expressed two antigen I/II polypeptides, SspA and SspB, products of tandem chromosomal genes (39).

Surface proteins of the antigen I/II family contain alanine-rich repeats, which adopt an a-helical coiled-coil structure, proline rich repeasts, and a carboxy-terminal region that includes the gram-positive cell wall anchor motif LPXTG (12, 49). Binding activity to salivary glycoprotein has been attributed to both the highly conserved alanine rich repeats (50, 51) and the proline-rich repeating sequences (52). In addition to salivary glycoprotein binding activity, SspA has been implicated in coaggregation of *S. gordonii* with Actinomyces (39). Such bacterial coaggregation may be involved in dental plaque formation.

Two other *S. gordonii* proteins, CshA and CshB, have also been implicated in coaggregation with Actinomyces. These adhesins may play a role in adherence of *gordonii* to immobilized fibronectin *in vitro* (52) and in colonization *in vivo* (40).

Staphylococcus aureus also expresses fibronectin-binding adhesins. Two genes encoding for fibronectin-binding proteins have been identified in *S. aureus fnb*A and *fnb*B (41). Fibronectin binding activity is critical in pathogenesis because it allows the bacteria to adhere to extracellular matrix components including fibornectin and collagen (53). This can result in cutaneous infections and in life-threatening bacteremia and endocarditis (54).

Binding to fibronectin is also essential for the attachment of *S. pyogenes* to respiratory endothelial cells. *S. pyogenes,* a group A streptococcus, has been implicated in various diseases from skin and throat infections to sepsis and shock (55). This binding activity is mediated by several fibronectin binding proteins. Six different genes encoding proteins with fibrollectin binding activity have been identified (12). The most well characterized are two closely related proteins, Sfbl (42) and Protein F (43). Both proteins are directly involved in the fibronectin mediated adherence to epithelial cells.

Another group of extensively studied streptococcal adhesins is the Lral family of proteins included in this group are FimA from *S. parasanguis*, PsaA from *S. pneumoniae*. ScaA from *S. gordonii*, ScbA from *S. crista*, SsaB from *S. sanguis*, and EfaA from *Enterococcus*

TABLE 5.2: Adhesins of Gram-positive Bacteria

Adhesion	*Strain*	*Ligand*	*Reference*
Antigen I/II Ag I/II, SpaP			Family Demuth (39)
Pl. PAc	*Streptococcus mutans*	Salivary glycoprotein	
SspA, SspB	*Streptococcus gordonii*	Salivary glycoprotein	
SpaA, P Ag	*Streptococcus Sobrinus*	Actinomyces Salivary glycoprotein	
CshA, CshB	*S. gordonii*	Actinomyces, Fibronectin	McNab (40)
FnbA, FnbB	*Staphylococcus aureus*	Fibronectin	Jonsson (41)
Sfbl. Protein F	*Streptococcus Pyogenes*	Fibronectin	Talay (42) Hånski (43)
Lral gamily			Burnett-Curley *et al.* (44)
Lral gamily			Jenkinson and Lamont (12)
FimA	*Streptococcus parasanguis*	Salivary glycoprotein fibrin	
PsaA	*Streptococcus Pneumoniae*	Unknown	
ScaA	*S. gordonii*	Actinomyces	
SsaB	*Streptococcus sanguis*	Salivary glycoprotein	
EfaA	*Enterococcus faecalis*	Unknown	
CbpA/SpsA/ PbwAc	*S. pneumoniae*	Cytokine activated	Rosenow (45) Hammerschmidt *et al.* (46)
PspC		Epithelial and Endothelial cells, 1gA	Briles *et al.* (47) Smith *et al.* (48)

faecalis (44.56). These membrane-bound lipoproteins are part of a larger family of ATP-binding cassette metal permeases, involved in the acquisition of manganese (57).

The adhesins FimA and SsaB have high affinity for salivary glycoprotein on tooth surfaces and are involved in colonisation of the oral cavity. The FimA adhesion for *S. parasanguis* has been localized to the tip of peritrichous surface fimbria on these bacteria (58). FimA is also a major virulence factor of *S. parasanguis* and binds fibrin (44).

The *S. pneumoniae* homologue of FimA. PsaA, also has a role in pathogenesis (59, 60). While it commonly colonizes the nasopharynx of healthy persons. *S. pneumoniae* is a common pathogen in children and older adults and a leading cause of otitis media, bacterial pneumonia, sepsis, and meningitis. Like its homologues. PsaA may function as an adhesin, according to initial evidence (61). Insertion inactivation of psaA resulted in pneumococcal mutants that exhibited reduced adherence to alveolar epithelial cells *in vitro* (60). However, the PsaA protein may be a permease involved in the regulation of adherence (57, 61).

Another pneumococcal protein thought to be an adhesin is CbpA (45) (also known as SpsA (46) and PspC (47), one of a family of choline binding proteins (CBPs) (*i.e.*, surface proteins noncovalently associated with the phosphocholine on the lipoteichoic acid). CbpA was initially isolated from a mixture of pneumococcal proteins that were able to bind to a choline affinity column. The CBP mix was purified from a strain with an inactivated pspA gene (45). The exogeneous CBP mix inhibited adherence of pneumococci to type II preumocytes and endothelial cells *in vitro*, suggesting that one or more of these proteins may act as adhesins, CbpA was the most abundant component in this mix and was shown to be on the surface of intact pneumococci in an indirect fluorescent labelling assay. The CbpA protein also reacted strongly with a pool of human convalescent phase serum. CbpA is thought to mediate adherence of *S. pneumoniae* to sialic acid and lacio-N-neutetraose ligands present on cytokine- activated epithelial and endothelial cells *in vitro* (45). In addition others have shown that this choline binding protein (which they called SpsA) has IgA-binding properties though the relevance of this function to pneumococcal pathogenesis is unclear (46).

Yet another group has demonstrated complement protein C3-binding activity for this protein, which they termed PbcA (48). Whatever its role in pathogenesis, we have demonstrated that the gene for CbpA (SpsA/PbcA/PspC) is highly conserved among the most common pneumococcal isolates, further enhancing its use as a vaccine candidate (62).

Bacterial Adhesins for Determinants of Microbial Colonisation and Pathogenicity

Bacterial adhesins are a critical determinant of microbial colonization and are fundamental to disease pathogenesis. No two adhesins are identical, reflecting the fact that each organism has a distinct ecological niche and is exposed to a different set of evolutionary pressures. Continued investigation is likely to identify additional paradigms and novel nuances (3).

The Mucosal Immune System for Fundamental Concepts to Vaccine Development

It is needed to develop fundamental concept of mucosal immune system for vaccine development. Recent studies in experimental animals and humans have shown that the mucosal immune system, which is characterized by secretary IgA (S-IgA) antibodies as the major humoral defence factor, contains specialized lymphoid tissues where antigens are encountered from the environment, are taken up and induce B-and T-cell responses. This event if followed by an exodus of specific lymphocytes, which home to various effect or sites such as the lamina propria regions and glands. These responses are regulated by T cells and cytokines and lead to plasma cell differentiation and subsequent production of S-IgA antibodies in external secretions. This knowledge has led to practical approaches from vaccine construction and delivery into mucosal inductive sites in an effort to elicit host protection at mucosal surfaces where the infection actually occurs (4).

Discussion

One of the key aspects of proving the potential efficacy of an adhesin-based vaccine *in vivo* is the development of an animal model of disease that relies on bacterial colonization of the mucosal epithelium mediated by the specific adhesin of interest. Although seemingly straightforward, testing for protection in small animal models of disease is difficult for various reasons like large doses of *in-vitro* grown bacteria are required to establish mucosal colonization in animals, which does not necessarily mimic the course of infection in humans; specific glycoprotein receptors for some adhesins are lacking in animal mucosal tissues that correspond to the site of colonization in humans; and some bacterial adhesins that are usually expressed as part of a larger structure on the bacterial cell surface (*e.g.* tip adhesins associated with whole pili) are difficult to purify. Despite these difficulties, adhesin-based vaccines have demonstrated efficacy in protecting against infection, thus proving the usefulness of such molecules as subunit vaccines.

Type 1 pili have long been implicated in bacterial urinary tract infections in humans (63, 64). In a murine cystitis model, colonization of the bladder by *E. coli* was shown to depend on growth conditions that favoured expression of type I pili and in particular required FimH (15, 65). Thus, the murine model was a valid small animal model to prove whether adhesin-based vaccines might block colonization.

Although purifying large amounts of pilus associated adhesin is difficult (because most adhesins are proteolytically degraded when expressed as independent moieties). Hultgren *et al.* (11) demonstrated that the FimH adhesin could be stabilized in an active conformation by the periplasmic chaperone FimC, making it possible to purify full-lengh FimH protein. Vaccination with the FimCH complex elicited long-lasting immune response to FimH. Sera from mice vaccinated with the FimH vaccine inhibited uropathogenic strains of *E. coli* from binding to human bladder cells *in vitro*. Vaccination with the FimH adhesin-vaccine reduced *in vivo* colonization of the bladder mucosa by >99 per cent in the murine cystitis model (15). Furthermore, the FimH vaccine protected against colonization and disease by uropathogenic strains of *E. coli* capable of expressing multiple adhesins. IgG specific for FimH was detected in the urine of protected mice, consistent with our original hypothesis that antibodies directed against an adhesin protein might protect along the mucosal surface. Subsequent studies in a primate model of cystitis have corroborated these findings (66). Furthermore, in primate studies we demonstrated a direct correlation between the presence of inhibitory antibodies in secretions and protection against colonization and infection.

While IgG antibodies elicited against adhesins are protective, induction of immune responses along the mucosa can be augmented by a variety of antigen delivery systems that specifically target mucosa-associated lymphoid tissue and activate the mucosal immune system (4-7, 67). These delivery systems include whole inactivated or live attenuated bacterial and viral vectors, biodegradable microspheres, liposomes, transgenic plants, and antigens conjugated to or coadministered with the cholera toxine B subunit or attenuated forms of heat labile toxin from *E. coli.* Many of these systems hold promise for future vaccine strategies, but only a few have been tested in humans for safety and adjuvanticity. As these mucosal adjuvants progress further toward approval for use in humans, testing should be done which adhesin antigens to determine if induction of local immune responses enhances the protective efficacy of adhesin-based vaccines as compared with conventional parenteral vaccination. Such studies are under way with the FimH vaccine.

Given the preclinical data with the FimH vaccine, similar efforts should be directed at developing adhesin based vaccines for a wide range of pathogens. In this regard, additional efforts should also be focussed on developing mucosal models of infection. The availability of such models should allow for appropriate screening of adhesin-based vaccines to prevent infections by streptococci, staphylococci, and other pathogens for which vaccine coverage may be inadequate.

Acknowledgement

In the preparation of this chapter help has been taken from various source papers which has been duly acknowledged. We are also grateful to Dr. Theresa M. Wizemann. Dr. John E. Adamou, and Dr. Solomon Langermann Medlmmune, Inc. Gaithersburg, Maryland, USA, for their kind help.

References

1. Hilleman, M.R. (1993). Paper presented at the International Symposium on Recombinant Vectors in Vaccine Development; 1993 May 23; Albany, New York. (Nucleic Acids Technologies Foundation, sponsored by IABS, FDA, USDN APHIS, and NIAID/NIH).

2. Alexander, J., Fikes, J., Hoffman, S., Franke, E., Sacci, J., Appella, E. Chisari, F. V., *et al.* (1998). The optimization of helper T

lymphocyte (HTL) function in vaccine development. *Immunol. Res.*, 18: 79-92.

3. St. Geme, J.W. III (1997). Bacterial adhesins: determinants of microbial colonization and pathogenicity. *Adv. Pediatr.*, 44: 43-72.
4. McGhee, J., Mestecky, J., Dertzbaugh, M.T., Eldridge, J.H., Hirasawa, M., Kiyono, H. (1992). The mucosal immune system: from fundamental concepts to vaccine development. *Vaccine*, 10: 75-88.
5. Langermann, S. (1996). New approaches to mucosal immunization. *Semin Gastrointest. Dis.*, 7: 12-18.
6. O'Hagan, D. T. (1998). Recent advances in vaccine adjuvants for systemic and mucosal administration. *J. Pharm. Pharmacol.*, 50: 1-10.
7. Mestecky, J., Michalek, S.M., Moldoveanu, Z., Russell, M.W. (1997). Routes of immunization and antigen delivery systems for optimal mucosal immune responses in humans. *Behring. Inst. Mitt.*, 98: 33-43.
8. Beachey, E.H. (1981). Bacterial-adherence: adhesin-receptor interactions mediating the attachment of bacteria to mucosal surface. *J. Infect. Dis.*, 143: 325-345.
9. Beachey, E.H., Giampapa, C.S., Abraham, S.N. (1988). Bacterial adherence: adhesin receptor mediated attachment of pathogenic bacteria to mucosal surfaces. *American Review of Respiratory Diseases*, 138: 545-548.
10. Ofek, I., Sharon, N. (1990). Adhesins as lectins: specificity and role in infection. *Curr. Top. Microbiol. Immunol.*, 151: 91-113.
11. Hultgren, S.J., Abraham, S., Capron, M., Falk, P., St. Geme, J.W., Normark, S. (1993). Pilus and non-pilus bacterial adhesins: assembly and function in cell recognition. *Cell*, 73: 887-901.
12. Jenkinson, H.F., Lamont, R.J. (1997). Streptococcal adhesion and colonization. *Crit. Rev. Oral. Biol. Med.*, 8: 175-200.
13. Abraham, S.N., Sun, D., Dale, J.B., Beachey, E.H. (1988). Conservation of the D-mannose-adhesion protein among type-I fimbriated members of the family Enterobacteriacaea. *Nature*, 682-684.

14. Sokurendo, E.V., Courtney, H.S., Ohman, D.E., Klemm, P., Hasty, D.L. (1994). FimH family of type I fimbrial adhesins: functional heterogeneity due to minor sequence variations among fimH genes. *J. Bacteriol.*, 176: 748-755.

15. Langermann, S., Palaszynski, S., Barnhart, M., Auguste, G., Pinkner, J.S., Burlein, J. *et al.* (1997). Prevention of mucosal *Escherichia coli* infection by FimH based systemic vaccination. *Science*, 276: 607-611.

16. Palaszynski, S., Pinkner, J., Leath, S., Barren, P., Auguste, C.G., Burlein, J. (1998). Systemic immunization with conserved pilus-associated adhesins protects against mucosal infections. *Dev. Biol. Stand.*, 92: 117-122.

17. Finlay, B., Falkow, S. (1989). Common themes in microbial pathogenicity. *Microbiological Review*, 53: 210-230.

18. Hoepelman, A.I., Tuomanen, E.I. (1992). Consequences of microbial attachment: directing host cell functions with adhesins. *Infect Immun*, 60: 1729-1733.

19. Svanborg, C., Hedlund, M., Connell, H., Agace, W., Duane, R.D., Nilsson, A. (1996). Bacterial adherence and mucosal cytokine responses: Receptors and transmembrane signalling. *Ann. N.Y. Acad. Sci.*, 797: 177-190.

20. Falkow, S. (1997). Invasion and intracellular sorting of bacteria: searching for bacterial genes expressed during host/pathogen interactions. *J. Clin. Invest.*, 100: 239-243.

21. Mecsas, J.J., Strauss, E.J. (1996). Molecular mechanisms of bacterial virulence: type III secretion and pathogenicity islands. *Emerg. Infect. Dis.*, 2: 270-288.

22. Zhang, J.P., Normark, S. (1996). Induction and gene expression in *Escherichia coli* after pilus-mediated adherence. *Science*, 273: 1234-1236.

23. Donnenberg, M.S., Kaper, J.B., Finlay, B.B. (1997). Interactions between enteropathogenic *Escherichia coli* and host epithelial cells. *Trends Microbiol.*, 5: 109-114.

24. Kenny, B., De, Vinney R., Stein, M., Reinscheid, D.J., Frey, E.A., Finlay, B.B. (1997). Enteropathogenic *E. coli* (EPEC) transfers its receptor for intimate adherence into mammalian cells. *Cell*, 91: 511-520.

25. Svanborg-Eden, C., Marild, S., Korhonen, T.K. (1982). Adhesion inhibition by antibodies. *Scand. J. Infect. Dis.*, 33: 72-78.

26. O'Hanley, P., Lark, D., Falkow, S., Schoolnik, G. (1985). Molecular basis of *Escherichia coli* colonization of the upper urinary tract in Balb/c mouse model of human pyclonephrities. *J. Clin. Invest.*, 75: 347-360.

27. Pecha, B., Low, D., O'Hanley, P. (1989). Gal-Gal pili vaccines prevent pyelonephritis by piliated *Escherichia coli* in a murine model. Single component Gal-Gal pili vaccines prevent pyelonephritis by homologous and heterologous piliated *E. coli* strains. *J. Clin. Invest.*, 83: 2102-2108.

28. Moon, H.W., Bunn, T.O. (1993). Vaccines for preventing enterotoxigenic *Escherichia coli* infections in farm animals. *Vaccine,* 11: 213-220.

29. Maurer, L., Orndorff, P. (1987). Identification and characterization of genes determining receptor binding and pilus length of *Escherichia coli* type I pili. *J. Bacteriol,* 169: 640-645.

30. Hanson, M.S., Brinton, C.C. Jr. (1988). Identification and characterization of the *Escherichia coli* type I pilus adhesin protein. *Nature,* 322: 265-268.

31. Bock, K., Breimer, M.H., Brignole, A., Hansson, G.C., Karisson, K.A., Larson, G. (1985). Specificity of binding of a strain of uropathogenic *Escherichia coli* to Gal 1-4Gal-containing glycosphingolipids. *J. Biol. Chem.*, 260: 8545-8551.

32. Stromberg, N., Marklund, B.I., Lund, B., Iiver, D., Hammers, A., Gaastra, W. (1990). Host specificity of uropathogenic *Escherichia coli* depends on differences in binding specificity to Gal 1-4 Gal-containing isoreceptors. *EMBO J.*, 9: 2001-2010.

33. Hulgren, S.J., Jones, C.H. (1995). Utility of the immunoglubulin-like fold of chaperones in shaping organelles of attachment in pathogenic bacteria. *American Society for Microbiology News*, 61: 457-464.

34. Brennan, M.J., Shahin, R.D. (1996). Pertussis antigens that abrogate bacterial adherence and elicit immunity. *Am. J. Respir. Crit. Care. Med.*, 154: 5145-5149.

35. St. Geme, J.W. III (1996). Progress towards a vaccine for nontypable Haemophilus influenzae. The Finnish Medical Society DUODECIM. *Ann. Med.*, 28: 31-37.

36. Barenkamp, S.J., St. Geme, J.W. III (1996). Identification of a second family of high-molecular weight adhesion proteins expressed by non-typable Haemophilus influenzae. *Mol. Microbiol.*, 19: 1215-1223.

37. Iiver, D., Amqvist, A., Ogren, J., Frick, I.M., Kersulyte, D., Incecik, E.T. (1998). Helicobacter pylori adhesin binding fucosylated histo-blood group antigens revealed by retagging. *Science*, 279: 373-377.

38. Roberts, J.A. (1996). Tropism in bacterial infections: urinary tract infections. *J. Urol.*, 156: 1552-1559.

39. Demuth, D.R., Duan, V., Brooks, W., Holmes, A.R., McNab, R., Jenkinson, H.F. (1996). Tandem genes encode cell surface polypeptides SspA and SspB which mediate adhesion of the oral bacterium *Streptococcus gordonii* to human and bacterial receptors. *Mol. Microbiol.*, 20: 403-413.

40. McNab, R., Jenkinson, H.F., Loach, D.M., Tannock, G.W. (1994). Cell-surface associated polypeptides CshA and CshB of high molecular mass are colonization determinants in the oral bacterium *Streptococcus gordonii. Mol. Microbiol.*, 14: 743-745.

41. Jonsson, K., Signas, C., Muller, H.P., Lindberg, M. (1991). Two different genes encode fibronectin binding proteins in *Staphylococcus aureus.* The complete nucleotide sequence and characterization of the second gene. *Eur. J. Biochem.*, 202: 1041-1048.

42. Talay, S.R., Valentin-Weigand, P., Timmis, K.N., Chhatwal, G.S. (1994). Domain structure and conserved epitopes of Sib protein, the fibronectin-binding protein adhesin of *Streptococcus pyogenes. Mol. Microbiol.*, 13: 531-539.

43. Hanski, E., Caparon, M., Protein, F. (1992). A fibronectin-binding protein, is an adhesin of the group A streptococcus, *Streptococcus pyogenes. Proc. Natl. Acad. Sci. USA*, 89: 6172-6176.

44. Burnette-Curley, D., Wells, V., Viscount, H., Munro, C.L., Fenno, J.C., Fives-Taylor, P. (1995). FimA, a major virulence factor associated with *Streptococcus parasanguis* endocarditis. *Infect. Immun.*, 63: 4669-4674.

45. Rosenow, C., Ryan, P., Weiser, J.N., Johnson, S., Fontan, P., Ortqvist, A. (1997). Contribution of novel choline-binding proteins to adherence, colonization and immunogenicity of *Streptococcus pneumoniae*. *Mol. Microbiol.*, 25: 819-829.

46. Hammerschmldt, S., Talay, S.R., Brandtzaeg, P., Chhatwal, G.S. (1997). SpsA, a novel pneumococcal surface protein with specific binding to secretarey immunoglobulin A and secretory component. *Mol. Microbiol.*, 25: 1113-1124.

47. Briles, D.E., Hollingshead, S.K., Swiatlo, E., Brooks-Walter, A., Szalai, A., Virolainen, A. (1997). PspA and PspC: their potential for use as pneumococcal vaccines. *Microb. Drug Resist.*, 1997: 3: 401-408.

48. Smith, D.L., Cheng, Q., Hostetter, M.K. (1998). *Characterization of a pneumococcal surface protein that binds complement protein C3 and its role in adhesion* (poster 6 D-122). The American Society for Microbiology 98th General Meeting; Atlanta, Georgia.

49. Hajishengallis, G., Russell, M.W., Michalek, S.M. (1998). Comparison of an adherence domain and a structural region of *Streptococcus mutans* antigen I/II in protective immunity against dental caries in rats after intranasal immunization. *Infect. Immun.*, 66: 1740-1743.

50. Crowley, P.J., Brady, L.J., Piacentini, D.A., Bleiweis, A.S. (1993). Identification of a salivary agglutinin-binding domain within cell surface adhesin PI of *Streptococcus mutans*. *Infect. Immun.*, 61: 1547-1552.

51. Todryk, S.M., Kelly, C.G., Lehner, T. (1998). Effect of route of immunisation and adjuvant on T and D cell epitope recognition within a streptococcal antigen. *Vaccine*, 16: 174-180.

52. McNab, R., Holmes, A.R., Clark, J.M., Tannock, G.W., Jenkinson, H.F. (1996). Cell surface potypeptide CshA mediate binding of *Streptococcus gordonii* to other oral bacteria and to immobilized fibronectin. *Infect. Immun.*, 64: 4202-4210.

53. Schennings, T., Heimdahl, A., Coster, K., Flock, J.I. (1993). Immunization with fibronectin binding protein from *Staphylococcus aureus* protects against experimental endocarditis in rats. *Microb. Pathog.*, 15: 227-236.

54. Lee, J.C. (1996). The prospects for developing a vaccine against *Staphylococcus aureus*. *Trends Microbiol.*, 4: 162-166.

55. Molinari, G., Talay, S.R., Valentin-Weigand, P., Rohde, M., Chharwal, G.S. (1997). The fibronectin binding protein of *Streptococcus pyogelles.* Sfbl. is involved in the internalization of group A streptococci by epithelial cells. *Infect. Immun.*, 65: 1357-1363.

56. Correla, F.F., DiRienzo, J.M., McKay, T.L., Rosan, B. (1996). schA from *Streptococcus crista* CCSA: an atypical member of the Iral gene family. *Infect. Immun.*, 64: 2114-2121.

57. Dintihac, A., Alloing, G., Granadel, C., Claverys, J.P. (1997). Competence and virulence of Streptococcus pneumoniae: Adc and PsaA mutants exhibit a requirement for An and Mn resulting from inactivation of putative ABC metal permeases. *Mol. Microbiol.*, 25: 727-739.

58. Fenno, J.C., Shaikh, A., Spatefora; G., Fices-Taylor, P. (1995). The fimA locus of *Streptococcus parasanguis* encodes an ATP-binding membrane transport system. *Mol. Microbiol.*, 15: 849-863.

59. Talkington, D.F., Brown, B.G. Tharpe, J.A., Koenig, A., Russell, H. (1996). Protection of mice against fatal pneumococcal challenge by immunization with pneumococcal surface adhesin A (PsaA). *Microb. Pathog.*, 21: 17-22.

60. Berry, A.M., Paton, J.C. (1996). Sequence heterogenity of PsaA, a 37-kilodalton putative adhesin essential for virulence of *Streptococcus pneumoniae. Infect. Immun.*, 64: 5255-5262.

61. Novak, R., Brown, J.S., Charpentier, E., Tuamonen, E. (1998). Penicillin tolerance genes of *Streptococcus pneumoniae:* the ABC-type marganese permease complex Psa. *Mol. Microbiol.*, 29: 1285-1296.

62. Dormizter, M., Wizemann, T.M., Adamou, J.E., Walsh, W., Gayle, T., Langermann, S. (1998). *Sequence and structural analysis of CbpA: A novel choline-binding protein of Streptococcus pneumoniae* (poster B-3). The American Society for Microbiology 98th General Meeting; Atlanta, Georgia.

63. Schaeffer, A.J., Amundsen, S.K., Schnidt, L.N. (1979). Adherence of *Escherichia coli* to human urinary tract epithelial cells. *Infect Immun.*, 24: 753-759.

64. Ofek, I., Mosek, A., Sharon, N. (1981). Mannose-specific adherence of *Escherichia coli* freshly excreted in the urine of

patients with urinary tract infections, and of isolates subcultured from the infected urine. *Infect. Immun.*, 34: 708-711.

65. Connell, H., Agace, W., Klemm, P., Schembri, M., Marild, S., Svanborg, C. (1996). Type I fimbrial expression enhances *Escherichia coli* virulence for the urinary tract. *Proc. Natl. Acad. Sci. USA*, 93: 9827-9832.
66. Wizermann, T.M., Adamou, J.E. and Langermann, S. (1999). Adhesins as Targets for Vaccine Development. *Emer. Infec. Dis.*, 5(3): 223-231.
67. Frey, A., Neutra, M.R. (1997). Targeting of mucosal vaccines to Peyer's patch M cells. *Behring Inst. Mitt.*, 98: 376-389.

CHAPTER 6

DEVELOPMENT FOR MALARIA NEW VACCINE A New Possibility for the World

Introduction

Every year 300 to 500 people affected by malaria. So, it is urgently needed to develop malarial vaccine, as vaccine are cost effective and easily administered. This chapter review efforts towards malarial vaccine development, observations that predict the success of malarial vaccine development, obstacles to vaccine development and possible vaccine for malaria.

It has been claimed that malaria continues an estimated about 3 million lives annually and to account for untold morbidity in the approximately 300-500 million people infected annually (1). Four species of protozoan parasites cause malaria in humans: *Plasmodium faiciparum, P, vivax, P. malariae* and *P. ovale. P. falciparum* is responsible for most deaths and most of the severe forms of disease, including cerebral malaria. At-risk groups include those in whom immunity has not yet developed (travellers, young children in endemic areas and so on) and those in whom immunity has diminished (pregnant women and people from endemic areas who have ceased to be routinely exposed to infection). Malaria is often cited as a substantial impediment to economic and social development in endemic regions.

Malaria is considered a re-emerging disease, mainly due to the spread of drug-resistant parasite strains, the decay of health-care infrastructure and difficulties in implementing and maintaining vector control programs in many developing countries and even US travellers and military or other personnel deployed in endemic areas. Each year there are more than 1,000 cases of 'imported' malaria reported in the US.

As a result of the spread of drug-resistant parasites and insecticide-resistant mosquitoes, in many respects there are now fewer tools to control malaria than existed even 20 years ago. Historically, vaccines have been one of the most cost-effective and easily administered means of controlling infectious diseases, and although no licensed vaccines exist against the disease, accumulating basic and clinical research suggests that they can be developed. This chapter review efforts towards malarial vaccine development, observations that predict the success of malarial vaccine development, obstacles to vaccine development and possible vaccine for malaria.

Efforts Towards Malarial Vaccine Development

Malaria parasites have complex life cycles associated with distinct developmental stages, each of which has multiple antigens that could serve as targets of an immune response. A pre-erythrocytic vaccine would protect against the infectious form injected by a mosquito (sporozoite) and/or inhibit parasite development in the liver. In a previously unexposed individual, if a few parasites were to escape the immune defenses induced by a pre-erythrocytic vaccine, they could eventually multiply and a result in full-blow disease. An erythrocytic or blood-stage vaccine would inhibit parasite multiplication in the red cells, thus preventing (or diminishing) severe disease during the blood infection. A sexual-stage vaccine does not protect the person being vaccinated, but instead interrupts the cycle of transmission by inhibiting the further development of parasites, once they-along with antibodies produced in response to the vaccine-are ingested by the mosquito. Transmission-blocking vaccines could be involved as part of a multi-faceted strategy directed to elimination of parasites from low-transmission areas or as a means of protecting a vaccine or drug directed at pre- erythrocytic or erythrocytic stages against the spread of resistant parasites. An optimal vaccine would have the ability to elicit protective immunity that blocks infection as well as prevents pathology and interrupts transmission of parasites, and would most likely be a combination vaccine composed of subunits from different parasitic stages.

Observations that Predict the Success of Malarial Vaccine Development

The following observations predict the eventual success of vaccine development for malaria:

1. Human populations residing in malaria endemic areas naturally acquire protective immunity.
2. Several studies show that immunoglobulin purified from the blood of immune adults from endemic regions can passively transfer protection against *P. falciparum*.
3. Clinical studies since the 1970s have demonstrated that experimental vaccination with attenuated sporozoites can effectively immunize patients against a subsequent malaria infection.
4. Animal models of malaria clearly substantiate the potential for induction of protective immunity with defined vaccines.

More than 30 distinct antigens identified in various life-cycle stages of the malaria parasite have been proposed, at some level, as potential vaccine candidates based on observations such as surface expression of the antigen on one or more life cycle stages *in vitro* inhibitory (invasion-blocking) effects of specific antibodies; or *in vivo* experiments showing protective effects of either direct immunization or passive transfer of antibody in animal models (2). Several early vaccine candidates, many based on the circumsporzoite (CS) protein, the dominant surface antigen of the sporozoite stage, progressed into Phase I/II clinical trials but were halted by problems of low immunogenicity and efficacy or, in some cases, by 'reactogenicity'.

Only one candidate vaccine, SPf66, based on antigens from both merozoite and sporozoite stages, has undergone extensive field trials. Efficacy was reported in several early clinical trials in South America, and one in Africa, but results from subsequent trials in Africa and Southeast Asia were not as promising (3, 4). Recent clinical studies of a vaccine composed of CS antigen and hepatitis B surface antigen (RTS, S) demonstrated that adjuvant is essential in successful immunization; these studies used the same antigenic construct with three different adjuvant formulations, only one of which induced significant protective immunity (5). These results emphasize the need not only to identify the right antigenic components for a vaccine, but also to find presentation and delivery methods that induce qualitatively and quantitatively appropriate immune responses.

So far, no pattern of immune response fully predictive of protection has been identified or validated. Naturally occurring immunity wanes rapidly in the absence of ongoing parasite exposure, and protection has been similarly short-lived in those few subunit vaccine trails that have demonstrated measurable efficacy. Such a vaccine might be useful for travellers. Unless new technologies can be found to improve the longevity of vaccine-induced resistance, however, it is likely that a vaccine to be used in endemic areas will need to take advantage of natural boosting provided by ongoing parasite exposure to provide long-lived protection.

In natural infection, unregulated immune responses may contribute to the pathogenesis of the disease. For example, an association of cerebral malaria with high plasma levels of pro-inflammatory cytokines has been reported (8). Thus, the potential for enhanced immunopathogenesls must also be taken into account in vaccine development efforts.

Experimental observations indicate that protective immunity may involve multiple different immune responses, both humoral and cellular (2, 6). The focus has been mainly on the induction of antibodies in the case of blood-stage and transmission blocking vaccines. Developers of pre-erythrocytic vaccines initially focused on induction of antibodies, then on CD8 + cytotoxic T lymphocytes (CTLs), and know additionally on T cell-derived cytokines. Interferon gamma (lFN-) and other cytokines seem to be involved in the elimination of liver stage parasites, possibly through induction of mediators such as nitric oxide that kill parasites within hepatocytes.

Obstacles to Malarial Vaccine Development

There are obviously many scientific questions that must be addressed in the course of further development efforts on malaria vaccines. These have been discussed at length elsewhere (2, 7) and include issues such as how to induce appropriate (protective, long-lasting, nonpathogenic) immune responses, how to structure combination vaccines, how to deal with parasite antigen diversity and antigenic variation, as well as how to deal with human genetic restriction of immune response and/or genetic predilection toward detrimental responses.

There are also a number of hurdles related to translational research and evaluation of candidate vaccines. These include issues regarding the appropriateness and accessibility of animal models. Other technical hurdles relate to the need to identity assays for on going validation of candidate antigens through process development and 'scale-up' production, as well as assays predictive of protection for the assessment of immunogenicity and efficacy in clinical trials. In addition, much careful thought must be given to clinical trial design. This is especially true for blood-stage vaccines, for which the leasibility of experimental challenge, infection is extremely controversial and the optimum measurement of efficacy is reduced morbidity/mortality, as well as for sexual-stage vaccines, for which the ultimate measurement of efficacy is interruption of malaria transmission (7).

It is anticipated that the scientific obstacles cited above can be overcome through research supported by expanded public-sector programs. Moreover, new or expanded public-sector programs have targeted one of the main logistic obstalcles cited in the 1993. Institute of Medicine report (7) that is, the requirement of cGMP production facilities for pilot lots of malaria antigens. The need remains, however, for help from the pharmaceutical and biotechnology industries resolving technical issues relating to appropriate expression and purification of antigens vaccine formulation and manufacturing technology. There can be no question that the dearth of committed industrial partners has limited progress in malaria vaccine development. The vaccine candidate that is now most advanced in clinical trials, RTS,S, has clearly benefited from the expertise provided by SBBio at all stages of this vaccine's research and development history. Likewise, other candidates have benefited greatly from partnerships with industry that provide access to proprietary technologies and reagents. These types of public-private-sector collaborations must be fostered, to overcome any perceived legal impediments.

In the 1996 Institute of Medicine report on *Vaccines against Malaria* (9), much emphasis was placed on the need for increased coordination of US governmental activities on malaria vaccine R and D to strengthen interactions with industry. Indeed, it is true that expanded efforts implemented since 1996 have mostly pursued parallel tracks within the different agencies (both in the US and other countries), and so far the number of potential vaccine candidates has clearly supported this approach. This parallelism may be further exacerbated with the predicted discovery of many more new malaria antigens through genomics research. Nonetheless, with limited resources for 'downstream' development priorities must eventually be identified. This would be greatly facilitated by mechanisms allowing for the development of combination vaccines, using antigens and/or adjuvants from different sources, as well as head-to-head comparisons of various candidates in preclinical and clinical trails. The identification of mechanisms to allow such sharing of proprietary reagents and information would contribute enormously to the rational development of malaria vaccines (10, 11).

Possible Vaccine for Malaria

The different types of possibility for malaria vaccines is following:

Approaches Towards Recombinant Vaccines

The Walter Reed Army Institute of Research (WEAIR) and Smith-Kline Beecham Biologicals (SBBio), through a 17-year partnership, are developing a multi-antigen, multi-stage malaria vaccine based on recombinant protein antigens. This collaboration has led to development of the CS-based RTS,S vaccine, which in combination with SBAS2 adjuvant repeatedly induced protection of volunteers in a Phase Iia trial. Subsesquent re-challenge of volunteers demonstrated that protection waned by months.

The first field trial of RTS,S/SBAS2, conducted by the Medical Research Council in The Gambia, reported 65 per cent efficacy in adult males in a region of intense transmission in which both homologous and heterologous *P. falciparum* strains are prevalent. Efficacy persisted for 2 months. The results from The Gambia further validate the standardized sporozoite challenge model used in Phase

FIGURE 6.1: Different Experimental Observations (for Vaccine Development) which may involve Multiple Different Immune Responses (Both Humoral and Cellular) that indicate Protective Immunity

Different Experimental Observations which may involve Multiple Different Immune Responses (Both Humoral and Cellular)

1. Antibodies to gametocytes, gametes or ookinetes can prevent development into sporozoites.
2. Antibodies to sporozoites can prevent invasion of hepatocytcs.
3. Inteferon gama and other cytokines can inhibit development of liver.
4. Cytoxic T lymphocytes can lyse infected hepatocytes.
5. Antibodies to merozoites can prevent invasion of erythrocytes.
6. Antibodies against parasite exoantiges may prevent induction of cytokinase pathway.
7. Antibodies to antigens on infected RBCs can eliminate the cells.
8. Cytokines can destroy the infected RBCs.

lia trials as a useful predictor of the efficacy of sporozoite-based vaccines in the field.

In partnership with SBBio, USAID, the Naval Medical Research Centre (NMRC) and others WRAIR is conducting preclinical, clinical and field trials to uptimize RTS, S/SBAS2 vaccine regimens; evaluate RTS,S with improved adjuvants; develop the blood-stage antigen merozoite surface protcin 1 (MSP1) as a potential component of a multi-stage, multi-antigen vaccine; and explore prime-boost strategies. Other WRAIR initiatives include development of the pre-erythrocytic liver-stage antigen I (LSA1), blood-stage antigens merozoite surface protein (FVO strain and 3D7 mutant) and apical membrane antigen I (AMA1), and attenuated venezuelan equine encephalitis virus as a platform for antigen delivery.

In a collaborative program between investigators at Oxford University and SBBio, detailed characterization of the cellular immune response to the RTS,S/SBAS2 vaccine is underway. Planned clinical trial include prime-boost studies of RTS,S boosted with a recombinant modified vaccinia virus ankara encoding the CS protein.

The NIAID Malaria Vaccine Development Unit (MVDU) is focusing on recombinant proteins derived from the blood and sexual stages of parasite development. Once produced and purified, blood-stage antigens are being tested in Aotus monkeys to identify the most promising candidates. Other aspects of the developmental pathway include the determination of optimal formulation in rhesus immunization studies, searching for immunologic assays that may correlate with protective immunity, exploration of synergistic responses to different parasite antigens and the execution of human clinical trials.

Blood-stage vaccines now being developed in the NIAID MVDU include the C-terminus of MSPI, and recent protection studies in the Aotus model system have shown promising results with a 42-kDa MSPI protein produced in baculovirus in collaboration with Novavax. A similar approach is also being tested by investigators at the University or Hawaii. A second candidate, PIEMPI, is expressed on the surface of infected red cells and thus is available to the immune system. A region of this variant parasite antigen that mediates binding of the infected cell to CD36 on vascular endothelial cells has shown promosing results in an Aotus trial. The MVDU is also conducting research on other blood-stage candidates, including MSP3, MSP4, MSP5 and AMAI. Transmission-blocking vaccines under development at the MVDU include Pfs25 and Pvs25, sexual stage (ookinete) antigens expressed by *P. falciparum* and *P. vivax*, respectively. Researcher at New York University are investigating the use of CS-based multiple antigenic peptides for induction of anti-sporozoite immunity. A synthetic multiple-antigenic-peptide vaccine containing minimal-T- and B-cell epitopes from the repeat region of the *P. falciparum* CS-protein with alum and QS21 elicited high levels of parasite-specific antibodies in a recent clinical trial, but immunogenicity was HLa-restricted. Newer methods for the synthesis of ple antigenic peptides and inclusion of universal epitopes are now being explored.

The CDC malaria vaccine program is focused on development of multi-valent, multi- stage vaccine formulations that contain a series of antigenic domains from all of the developmental stages of the parasite. This strategy, which is aimed at inducing 'multiple layers' of long-lasting, effective immunity, takes into consideration the immunogenicity and genetic diversity of antigenic fragments contained in stage- specific proteins, Two *P. falciparom* candidate vaccines are being investigated. One, a protein of 41 kDa called FALVAC-1, contains 21B- and T-cell epitopes from a variety of pre-erythrocytic, erythrocytic and sexual stages: CS,LSA1 , MSP1, SSP2, MSP2, AMA1, rhoptry-associated protein 1 (RAP1), EBA-175 and Pfg27, FALVAC-1 has been expressed in a baculovirus expression system, and mouse, rabbit and monkey immunization studies with various adjuvants demonstrated induction of immune responses that recognize different stages of the parasite.

A second candidate, FALVAC-2, containing the 19-kDa fragment of MSPl, the third epidermal growth factor domain of Pfs25, region II of EBA-175, as well as 30 B-cell epitopes and 25 T-cell epitopes from a total of 13 stage-specific antigens, is being developed. Similar approaches are underway for the development of multi-valent, multi-stage *P. vivax* vaccines. The goal for the next 5 years is to test multi-valent, multi-stage *P. falciparum* and *P. vivax* recombinant vaccines in non-immune persons and individuals living in malaria endemic areas.

The Australian malaria vaccine program is developing prototype asexual stage vaccines based on the 190L fragment of MSP1, MSP2, the ring-associated surface antigen RESA, AMA1, RAP1 and RAP2. Five human vaccine trials have been conducted with combinations of recombinant MSP1, MSP2 and RESA in the Montanide ISA 720 adjuvant (SEPPIC). In test animals, including monkeys, AMA1 and RAP2 have given very encouraging protection. The first Phase I human trial has been conducted with AMA1, further Phase I trials with AMA1 and RAP2 and planned for later this year.

Approaches Towards DNA Vaccine and Prime-boost

The Naval Medical Research Center (NMRC), in collaboration with Vical, USAID, Aventis Pasteur, Entremed and many investigators around the world, has initiated a DNA-based malaria vaccine development effort called the 'Multi-Stage DNA Vaccine Operation or MuStDO'. The goal during the next 3-4 years is to assess a 5-gene pre-erythrocytic stage vaccine (MuStDO 5) and a 15-gene pre-erythrocytic plus erythrocytic stage vaccine (MuStDO 15) as DNA vaccines alone, and as the priming component of a prime-boost regimen with recombinant protein in adjuvant and recombinant viruses as the boosters. These studies are ultimately aimed at assessing the capability of the vaccines to prevent blood-stage infection entirely in native individuals visiting highly endemic areas of Africa, and to prevent death in infants and young children in Africa. So far, initial Phase I studies in the US using a single-gene *P. falciparom* CS DNA vaccine have established safety as well as immunogenicity for CD8 + CTLs as well as CD8 + and CD4 + IFN-g-producing cells. In May 2000, a Phase I/Iia study will be initiated in which the 5-gene vaccine will be given with and without a plasmid expressing the cytokine granulocytemonocyte colony-stimulating factor to enhance immunogenicity.

Researchers at Oxford are assessing the safety, immunogenicity and efficacy of a DNA prime-MVA (modified vaccinia Ankara) boost regime in healthy volunteers. The insert, which is the same in the DNA and the MY A components, is a polyepitope string fused to the entire TRAP antigen (thrombospondin-related anonymous protein, also known as sporozoite surface protein 2, or SSP2, which is expressed mainly by spprozoites and liver-stage parasites). The delivery of DNA by an intramuscular route and by a needle-less delivery device into the skin is being compared. MVA is delivered intradermally. Initial studies of both DNA and MVA vaccines established adequate safety and immunogenicity. The first prime-boost studies of volunteers were initiated in December 1999 and are ongoing, with challenge studies anticipated later this year. Plans are underway to test both DNA and MVA vaccines in The Gambia in late 2000.

Approaches Towards Transgenic Vaccines

Genzyme Transgenics and the NIAID have established a collaboration for preclinical development of an MSP1-based vaccine in transgenic animals. The 42-kDa fragment of MSP1 has been produced in milk of transgenic mice, and a purification process is now being developed. If the purified product can be shown to protect Aotus monkeys, it will provide supporting data supporting the development of other transgenic animals such as goats.

Approaches Towards Genomic and Bioinformatics

In 1996, a collaborative international effort was undertaken to sequence the complete genome of *P. falciparum*. So far, two of the parasite's fourteen chromosomes have been completely sequenced and the sequences of many of the remaining chromosomes are nearing completion.

Although there have been substantial technical hurdles in sequencing this AT-rich organism, it is now estimated that essentially all of the parasite's approximately 6,000 genes are available in existing databases.

Thus the malarial community and vaccine developers have access to almost all of the genes encoding the antigens and proteins expressed by this organism, Although not validated, computer algorithms are being conceived to identity genes whose expressed products are potential candidate vaccine antigens by virtue of their predicted cell surface localization, stage-specific expression or structural features that may interact with components of the human host's immune system to initiate a protective response. Accompanying the development of such computational methods are high-throughput methods (DNA chips and microarrays, and proteomics) of differential gene and protein expression to identity and characterize antigens that may be appropriately exposed to the immune system. A challenge for malaria investigators is the limiting amounts of material available for certain stages of the parasite's life cycle, especially the liver stages.

In addition to the targeted and rational approaches described above, investigators are developing high-throughput 'shotgun' methods for candidate vaccine identification. For example, studies are underway to immunize mice with expression libraries prepared in genetic immunization vectors to help identify candidate vaccines in an unbaised, systematic manner using the *P. yoelii* rodent model of malaria.

The human genome project is providing immunologists with access to all of the immune response genes. It is anticipated that future developments will enable the investigators to determine the expression of all of these genes on chips and microarrays from large numbers of individuals. Analysis of gene expression from these individuals should lead to identifying immune correlates of protection and disease. Moreover, such methods will prove useful in studies of vaccine efficacy and safety.

Conclusion

The need for enhanced public-private-sector collaboration to support development of new public health tools for 'orphan' diseases such as malaria has been emphasized repeatedly in number of ways over recent years. The US government has also shown interest in the development of new mechanisms for pursuing this goal for development of a challenge grant program at the NIH to promote joint ventures with biotechnology, pharmaceutical and medical device industries.

This is a very opportune moment to explore methods to eliminate impediments to collaboration and put these much-needed partnerships in place. So, it is needed to take then challenges by the government agencies and pharmaceutical companies, simultaneously in both the developing and developed countries for the discovery, development and testing of new malaria vaccine candidates to emancipate a huge global population from the dreadful disease that exhibits a tendency of re-emergence in the different parts of the world.

Acknowledgement

In the preparation of this chapter help has been taken from various source papers which has been duly acknowledged. We are also grateful to Dr. Stephanie James and Dr. Louis Miller National Institute of Allergy and Infectious Diseases, National Institutes of Health, Bethesda, Maryland, USA, for their kind help.

References

1. Weekly Epidemiological Record of the World Health Organization (1996). 71: 17.
2. Hoffman, S.L. (Ed.) (1996). *Malaria Vaccine Development: A Multi-immune Response Approach.* ASM, Washington DC.
3. Miller, L.H. and Hoffman, S.L. (1998). Research towards vaccines against malaria. *Nature Med.*, 5: 520.
4. Facer, C.A. and Tanner, M. (1997). Clinical trials of malaria vaccines: progress and prospects. *Adv. Parasitol.*, 39: 1.
5. Stoute, J.A. (1997). A preliminary evaluation of a recombinant circumsporozoite protein vaccine against *Plasmodium falciparum* malaria. *N. Engl. J. Med.*, 336: 86.

6. Good, M.F. and Doolan, D.L. (1999). Immune effector mechanisms in malaria. *Curr. Opin. Immunol.*, 11: 412.
7. (1991). *Malaria: Obstacles and opportunities.* National Academy, Washington, DC.
8. Riley, E.M. (1999). Is T-cell, priming required for initiation of pathology in malaria infections? *Immunol. Today*, 20: 228.
9. (1996). *Vaccines against malaria: Hope in a gathering Strom.* National Academy, Washington, DC.
10. James, S. and Miller, L. (2000). Malaria vaccine development: Status report. *Nature Medicine.*
11. Dorin, D., Roch, K. Le., Sallicandro, P., Alano, P., Parzy, D., Poullet, P., Meijer, L., and Doerig, C., Pfnek-1, (2001). A NIMA-related kinase from the human malaria parasite *Plasmodium falciparom;* Biochemical properties and possible: involvement in MAPK regulation. *Eur. J. Biochem.*, 268: 2600-2608.

CHAPTER 7

Computer Aided Drug Designing

Introduction

At present, searches are being made to accelerate the designing of new drugs and at the same time to considerably reduce the associated expenses. The process of designing a new drug generally consists of 3 stages: (1) search for a new agent having the required pharmacological activity; (2) experimental studies and pharmacological and toxological tests; (3) all appropriate pharmacological committee's approval for clinical tests of the agent. Stage I is the most expensive and labour-consuming, as it requires a half the total expenditures. Its clinical version consists in the synthesis of numerous homologues of the well-known biologically active compounds and in long-term and costly trials. At the same time, an investigator has a definite range of concepts of the structure of a new drug as a new representative of the known group that he already knows. The application of computer-aided analysis and design enables these disadvantages to be overcome. The introduction of methods for pre-designing computer-aided drug design has permitted drastic reduction of expenses and accelerated designing of new drugs, by decreasing the number of unsuccessful syntheses and trials.

In the beginning, plants and other natural products were the source of most medicinal substances. For example, the foxglove plant can be used to treat congestive heart failure. As the science of medicinal chemistry evolved, it was discovered that foxglove contains digitalis and other cardiotonic glycosides which are responsible for the therapeutic effect. It became possible to isolate the active components, so that dosage could be more accurately regulated. Other medicines came about because of accidental observations and discoveries. Pencillim is one good example. Alexander Fleming noticed that some of his bacterial cultures were ruined because of contamination with mold. Wherever the mold grew, the bacteria were apparently killed. It was found that the mold (Penicillium) produces a substance called penicillin, which kills many kind of bacteria.

The discovery of penicillin led to a large-scale screening effort, in which thousands of soil microorganisms were grown and tested to see whether they could produce other substances which kill bacteria. Antibiotics such as streptomycin, neomycin, gentannicin, erythromycin, and the tetracyclines results from these efforts.

Chemical modification of known drugs can often lead to improved drugs. Naturally occurring penicillin G (below left) is broken down by bacterial beta-lactamases. Addition of two-OCH3 groups produces methicillin (below right), which is resistant to lactamase. Another example of chemical modification: opiate analgesics. The parent compound is morphine, which occurs in opium poppies. Morphine is a powerful analgesic, but it has serious side effects: respiratory depression, constipation, and dependence liability. Thousands of analogs (related chemical structures) have been synthesized in an effort to find analgesics with lower incidence of side effects. In some cases, small changes in chemical structure may have a big influence on the activity: nalorphine is a partial agonist (show some morphine-like activity, and at higher concentration, antagonizes morphine effects), and naloxone is an antagonist. Considerable simplification of the molecule is possible. Meperidine has only two rings instead of four, but it maintains strong analgesic activity. It has better oral absorption than morphine, and shows less Gl side effects. Methadone is an analgesic in which the original piperidine ring (6-membered ring containing a nitrogen atom) is completely absent. It retains analgesic activity, has good oral activity, and has a long half-life in the body. Dextromethorphan is constructed on a mirror-image of the morphine ring system. It has no opiate analgesic effects or side effects, but is a useful anti-tussive agent.

But today one of the most promising applications of this biologically based computer technique is in computer-aided molecular design (CAMD). This field has been called many things in different disciplines, but in general, it is the design of new molecules based on desired properties. In pharmaceutical development, this effort is focused on modelling the drugs and the biological receptors that the drugs bind to the specific site so that better binding, and therefore, more potent or precise drugs, can be developed (1). Evolutionary techniques can help achieve the design of totally new molecules, some that were never even thought of before.

Before evolutionary techniques can be applied in CAMD, two things must be known to some extent: the properties that are desired and how they relate to a molecule's structure. The structure-activity relationship is needed to determine the necessary properties and also build a molecule that has been endowed with those properties. This can be described as a structure-to-property stage and a property-to-structure stage (Figure 7.1). The first stage is determining the properties of a molecule based on its structure. The second stage is building a structure based on desired properties.

It's like telling a team of car engineers to build a better car. First, the aliens must figure out what a car does and how it works, and then they can build a new one based on what was learned.

Structure-to-Properties

The first stage, originally called the "forward problem" as conceived by Venkat enkatsubramanian of Purdue University, USA is essential for designing molecules by computer. Early attempts at approximating the properties of a molecule based on structure were successful for compounds with properties that varied in a direct way from their structure. However, this relationship soon becomes non-linear as more complicated molecules are modelled (2).

Pharmaceutical drug development using computer design techniques inherently requires complex molecular modelling. Drugs, or ligands, vary from the simple to the complex, but the receptors are usually extremely complex. Drug development is further complicated by the fact that it is a bimolecular system composed of the biological receptor and the ligand (drug or protein). Many CAMD systems choose to predict the properties of either the ligands that operate on the receptor or the receptor itself, but not usually both (3-7).

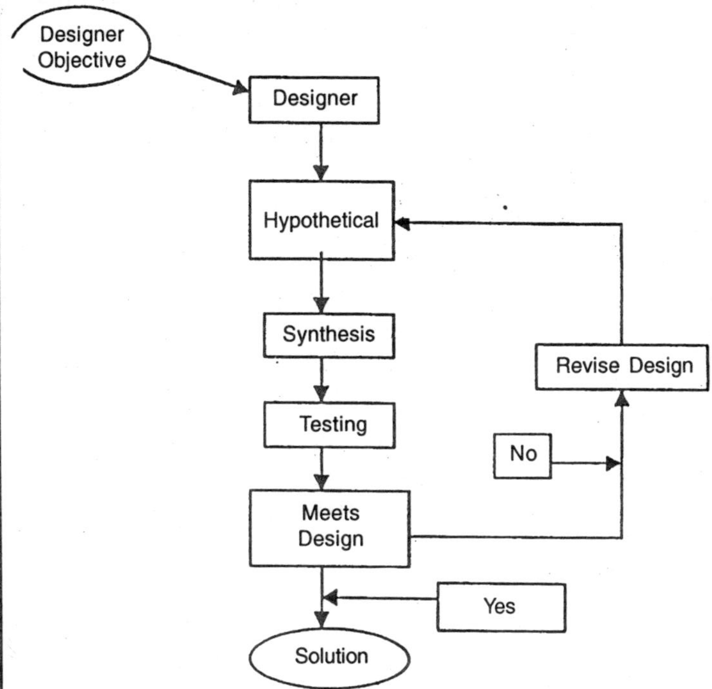

FIGURE 7.1: Process for Iterative Molecular Design

Systems that depend on the structure of a biological receptor face extreme difficulties. Many receptors are membrane-bound, making it extremely difficult to determine their three-dimensional structure by NMR or X-ray crystallography. Only a few thousand receptors are found in the protein data banks, and the structures may be based on the receptor being in water or organic solvents, which may prove to be an incorrect assumption. To complicate matters further, receptors may change shape as they bind a process called induced fit. If this is the mechanism of how a receptor and ligand bind, then the three-dimensional structure of the unbound receptor may be of slim relevance. Three-dimensional structure can be produced in which the receptor is bound to the ligand, however, this adds significant time and complexity to the procedure.

In addition to the difficulties facing the determination of structures, the shortcomings of computational modelling abilities are apparent for both receptors and ligands.

According to a patent from Axys Pharmaceuticals, Inc. (U.S. Patent 6081766; 2000), "Existing methods for constructing predictive models are unable to model steric interactions accurately, particularly when these interactions involve lare regions of the molecular surface". Likewise, quantitative structure-activity relationship (QSAR) techniques are rather accurate on a small scale, determining properties of specific regions but failing to produce all accurate global description of the molecule. Substituent models also incur problems when used on a different base molecule than the one for which the empirical data were measured (8-10).

If functional areas that might participate in binding are identified with QSAR properties, then those regions can be weighed heavily in determining the molecule's activity. This is a pharmacophore and can be used to characterize the whole molecule. Pharmacophore models attempt to combine some of the advantages of QSAR techniques with the idea of identifying substituents (11-13).

Although the above descriptions show many possible shortcomings of the present techniques, advances in three-dimensional QSAR have led to better characterization of molecules and better calculation of their properties. Increases in computer power allow more data points to be generated for surface properties, making the current field of functions closer estimations of macroproperties than ever before.

Properties-to-Structure

The second half of the challenge in developing a new molecule is to take the properties that you know are important and determine the structure that will have them. This has proven much more difficult than it sounds, and it depends on the first structure-to-properties part.

Various computational techniques have been used in the past to develop structures, but many have been unsuccessful. Both strictly computational and rule-based equations have encountered difficulty. These techniques "suffer from drawbacks due to combinational complexity of the search space, design knowledge acquisition difficulties, non-linerstructure-property correlations, and problems incorporating higher-level chemical and biological knowledge." The difficulties that scientists face in using these mathematical and reason-based methods have led to the search for better methods of developing new structures (18-24).

Criteria of Drug Designing Through Evolutionary Computing

The use of evolutionary techniques to create new molecules from properties largely reduces the difficulties presented by other methods of assembly. In general, two functions are used together to generate the evolutionary technique; genetic algorithms and fitness functions. Genetic algorithms produce mutations and crossover, something like sexual reproduction, to produce new species of data. The fitness function rounds out the evolutionary system by testing all the data and eliminating the poor performers, just like survival of the fittest.

For survival of fittest drug design, a new drug must satisfy several criteria:

1. Be safe to use
2. Be effective for the intended use
3. Be stable (chemically and metabolically)
4. Have a good solubility profile
5. Be synthetically feasible
6. Be novel (patentable)

Safe

All drugs have side effects. Drug designer have a large therapeutic index, the ratio between the toxic dose and the therapeutic dose. It is needed to start with acute toxicity tests in mice and to check for mutagenicity and teratogenicity, chronic effects over several generations. Safety tests is needed in several species of animals before the trial of the same on humans. It is also needed careful monitoring of adverse reactions in all phases of clinical trials. In the U.S., there are three phases of clinical trials.

In Phase I, the compound is tested in healthy volunteers at a range of doses to establish that there are no immediate adverse effects.

In Phase II, the compound is rested in a small number of patients in order to establish that there is an effect and to find what dosage may be required to achieve this effect.

In Phase III, large scale double-blind trials are carried out. Usually the compound is compared to an established drug or to placebo. This allows an objective measure of the drug's effectiveness.

And after approval, there is continued monitoring for adverse effects. This is sometimes referred to as "Phase IV". The drug can get stalled fore more testing.

Effective

This is the obvious one. But it's not cheap. One have to do some son of screening to identify the active compounds. Designer has to do some *in vivo* testing in animals to show that it works. Designer has to do lots of animal studies before he can try it out in humans. Then have to go through Phase I, Phase II, and Phase III clinical trials, send the paperwork to FDA, and wait for approval. Each stage gets progressively more expensive. Your drug candidate can fail to move along at any of these stages.

Stable

Chemical stability is absolutely for the drug under reference necessary. Aspirin breaks down over a period of time when exposed to humidity [sniff an old bottle to see if one can detect the acetic acid (vinegar) odor]. Designer need to do stability testing on his dosage form so that he can put a reasonable expiry date on it. Chemical stability also extends to the acid environment of the stomach for oral medications.

Metabolic stability is also important. Will the drug survive the various metabolic enzymes of the GI tract? If not, it is needed to use a parenteral dosage form. Will the drug be rapidly destroyed in the liver? Will it induce liver enzymes which affect the breakdown of other drugs, causing drug interactions?

Soluble

How water-soluble is the drug? Designer will need at least some water-solubility in order to get absorption and distribution of the drug throughout the body. But if it's too water-soluble, it will rapidly leave via the kidneys.

Lipid-solubility is also important. If the lipid-solubility is very low, the drug will not be absorbed well across lipid membranes. If it is too lipid-soluble, it may partition into fat stores and not reach the intended site of action.

The balance between these two properties is measured roughly by the octanol-water partition coefficient. When octanol and water are mixed, they form a two-phase system (like an oil-and vinegar dressing). Octanol roughly approximates the hydrophobicity of membrane lipids. So snake the drug in a mixture of octanol and water, let the layers separate, and measure the amount of the drug in each layer. The ratio (conc. in octanol) / (conc. in water) is the partition coefficient, P. The logarithm of P (log P) should ideally be less than S.

Synthetically Feasible

It's one thing for a chemist to spend six months in a lab to make 10 mg of a compound to test. But when company is going to market with a new drug. Designer has to be able to make it in kg quantities. This means it can't be a 14-step procedure, it can't use exotic solvents/reaction conditions, and starting materials must be readily available cheaply, in large quantity. If it's going to high cost, designer won't sell very many.

Novel

The drug has to be sufficiently novel that designer can patent it. Designer need patent protection in order to justify the $100 million designer will spend to get approval for the drug. And it has to be sufficiently novel that it doesn't infringe someone else's patent.

Computer-Aided Molecular Design Using Genetic Algorithms

Genetic algorithms (Gas) allow computers to generate new, random data (14-17). When combined with a fitness function, only the best data are randomly exchanged and mutated until a new generation of data is produced. As with real genes, genetic algorithms manipulate so-called genetic, material, but instead of DNA, this genetic material is some other linear string of symbols. In humans, the genetic material is DNA, which is thought of in terms of its base pairs. A string of three base pairs makes up a codon, which indicates the placement of a specific amino acid within a protein. By analogy, the computer equivalent of the base pairs and codon is replaced with a symbol or numbers that can represent any structural unit. For instance, a researcher might want to alter the molecular structure of a small molecule and could use symbols to represent the atoms or functional groups of potential molecules (25-28). Then N could indicate a nitrogen atom, or (Carb) could stand for a carboxylic acid group. Often, to promote faster computing, larger units are used, like replacing atoms with functional groups rather than adding all the complexity of the entire structure.

When genetic algorithms (GA) techniques are used the genetic material used is often different for different researchers or companies. One company may use number to designate substituent groups so mutations would change what substituents are used. Other may use letters to indicate molecular properties, such as saying P represents a region that is partially positive, and N represents something that is partially negative. Different GA techniques use different methods to convert the data into suitable genetic material; however what happens to the material is consistent (29-38).

The GA causes either mutation, crossover, or both. Mutation is the random changing of individual genetic symbols. For example, a string HGTZREU could have a GA that changes the R to a Q, and the new molecule would then be measured by the fitness function. Crossover is analogous to sexual reproduction, but it is a much cruder version. The GA randomly cuts the string of two different individuals in two, as seen in Figure 7.3. The half strings then switch so that there are two progeny, each with half from the parent. The children and the parents are then evaluated by the fitness function: the successful progeny and parents go on to be manipulated again by the GA (39-51).

In addition to Gas, there are different genetic programs that operate on data in a tree format, and genetic graphs, which are based on graph theory. Figures 7.4 and 7.5 illustrate the use of genetic programs and genetic graphs on molecules. Graph data for molecules is composed of a group of atoms-the vertices–that are held together by bonds, which are known as edges. Globis (12) at the National Aeronautics and Space Administration have tested this system against a set of already known compounds, including cholesterol, morphine, and diazepam.

The problem of designing new molecules with desired properties is obviously important, encompassing the design of polymers, polymeric composites, blends, paints and varnishes, refrigerants, solvents, drugs, pesticides, and so on. The traditional approach to this problem often requires a search involving a combinatorially large number of potential candidate molecules. It is an expensive and time-consuming iterative process with the scientist or engineer hypothesizing a compound, synthesizing the material, testing for desired properties, and redesigning the candidate if the desired properties are not met (Figure 7.1).

Computer-aided molecular design (CAMD) is an attractive alternative to the traditional synthesize and test methodology. The CAMD approach requires the solution of two problems (Figure 7.2): the forward problem requires the computation of macrosropic properties given the molecular structure, while the backward problem required the identification of the appropriate molecular structure given the desired problem; however, there has been considerably less progress in the backward problem which poses a real challenge for CAMD. Even though some researchers had addressed the backward problem using an enumeration approach some time back, Gani and Brignole, 1983 (11), Derringer and Markham, 1985 (8), major attention was drawn to this design problem by the important contribution of Joback and Stephanopoulos (1989) (29) recently, who proposed a heuristicsguided enumeration technique to combat the combinatorial complexity of molecular design. Subsequently, mathematical programming (29) and knowledge-based approaches have also been proposed by Nagasaka *et al.*, 1990 (30), Gani *et al.*, 1991(13). While all these methodologies have certain appeal and advantages, they also suffer from some serious drawbacks. For complex and industrially relevant molecules, these approaches have limitations due to combinatorial complexity, non-linear search spaces with local minima traps, difficulties in knowledge acquisition, difficulties in dealing with the non-linear structure-property correlations, and problems in incorporating higher level chemical knowledge and reasoning strategies. Thus, there exists a critical need to explore alternate strategies for molecular design that can circumvent these problems.

This chapter describes a novel framework for computer-aided molecular design using *Genetic Algorithms* (GA) to address these

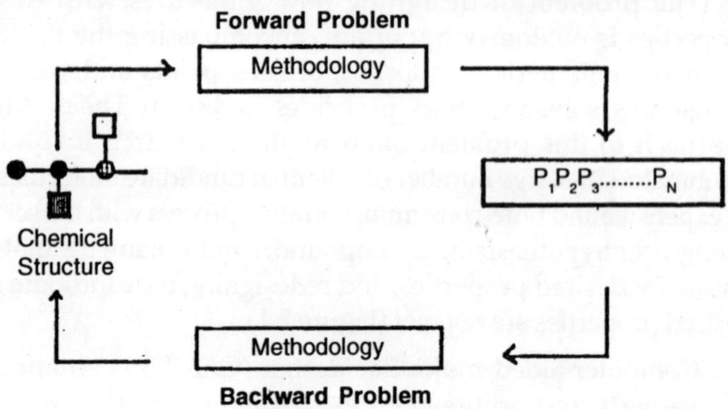

FIGURE 7.2: Components of the Molecular Design Problem

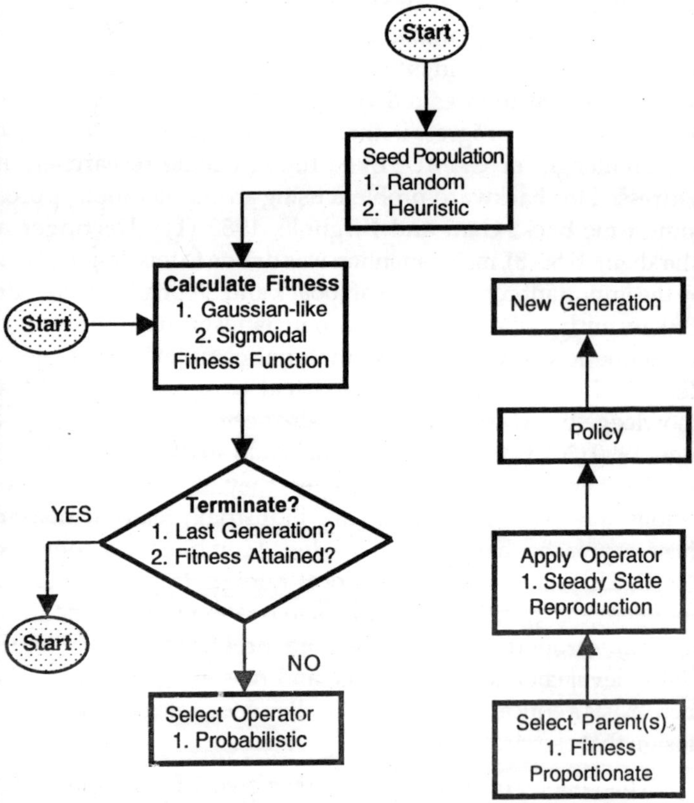

FIGURE 7.3: Genetic Algorithm Framework for CAMD

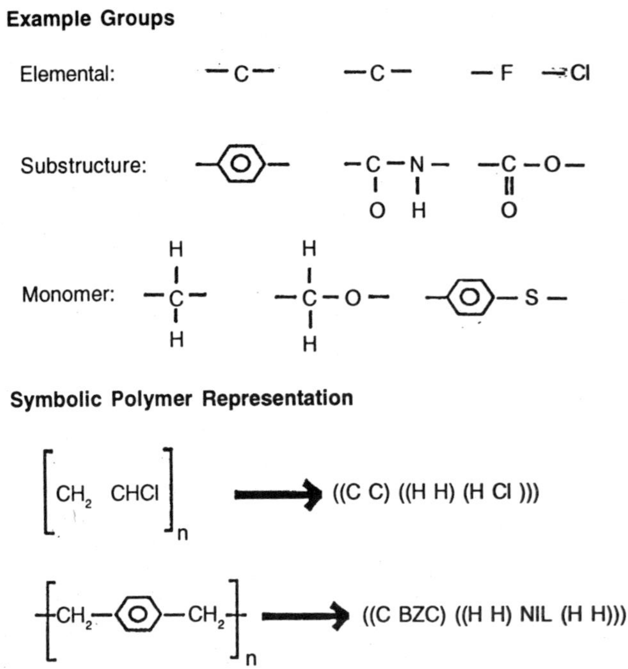

FIGURE 7.4: Molecular Structure Representation

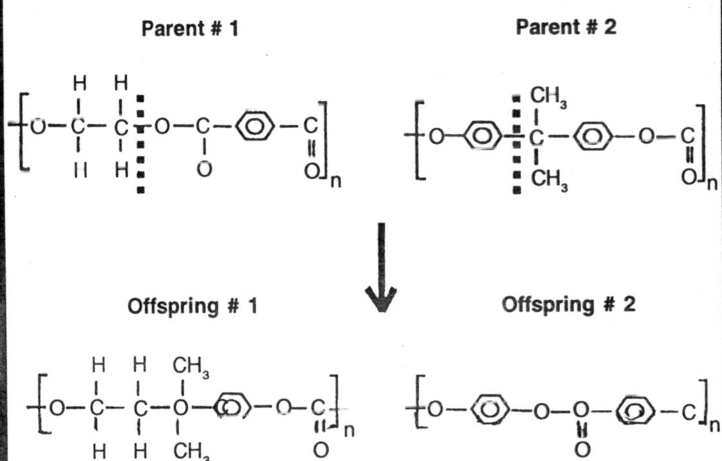

FIGURE 7.5: One-point Crossover Operator

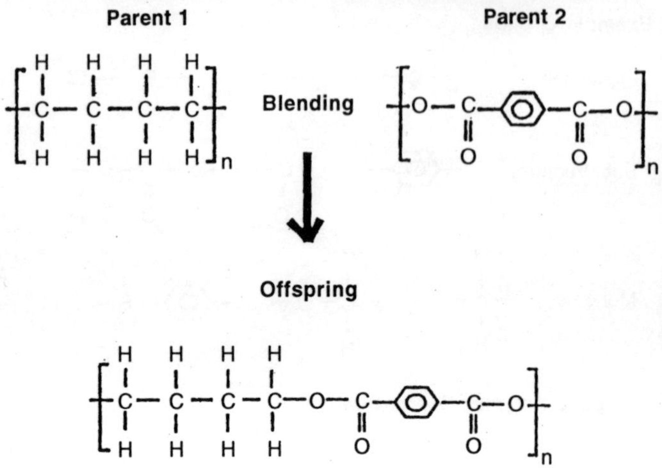

FIGURE 7.6: Blending Operator

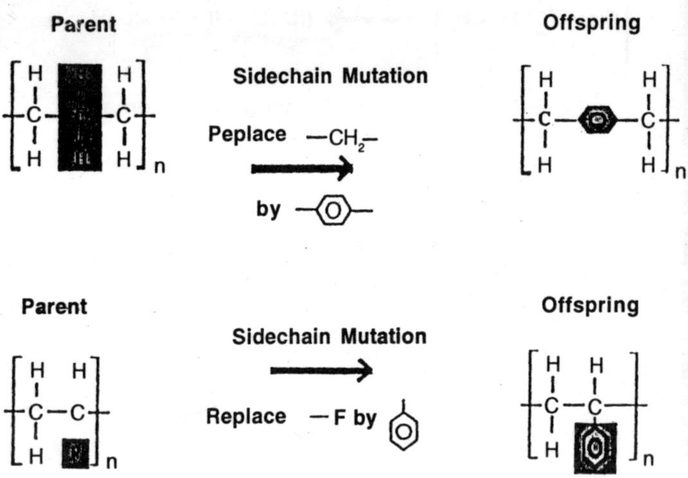

FIGURE 7.7: Mainchain and Sidechain Mutation Operators

limitations. The proficiency with which genetic algorithms are known to search noisy, discontinuous, and non-convex solution spaces motivated us to examine the genetic search as a viable framework for molecular design followed by Venkatasubramanian *et al.*, 1994 (45). In the rest of the chapter, we first discuss the important aspects of our genetic algorithmic approach, such as molecular representation, genetic operators, fitness functions, etc. This is followed by results from some case studies in polymer design which is showed by Venkatasubramanian *et al.*, (1995) (46) later we conclude with a discussion.

Genetic Algorithms for Evolutionary Creation

Genetic search methods have their basis in Darwinian model of natural selection and evolution. Introduced by Holland (1975) (16), the general idea behind genetic algorithms is the evolutionary creation of a new population of entities from an earlier generation through crossover and mutation processes and by passing on the fittest offsprings to the next generation. In general this approach is ultimately expected to lead to generations that become more and more fit through evolution thus achieving the desired design objective. However, there is no guarantee that this would be achieved, which is the primary drawback of the genetic search.

There are essentially two main components in a genetic algorithm. First, there must be a code or structure to represent the possible solutions to the problem. This basis code is called a *string*. Strings are composed of a sequence of characters of finite length n, composed of binary bits or symbols. Each candidate solution is represented by such a string. The set of solutions, Pj, is referred to as the *population* of the jth generation. Second, a transition rule must be defined to mimic the biological evolution process. The transition rule consist of a *reproductive plan* and *genetic operators*. The reproductive plan is an algorithm that select strings of the current population, which will participate in the process of generating the next solution population. The genetic operators appropriately modify the structure of the selected strings, in order to produce the members of next generation. A simple genetic algorithm consists of one reproductive plan, called the *fitness proportionate reproduction* and two genetic operators, *crossover* and *mutation* (Goldberg, 1989) (14).

In fitness proportionate reproduction, the probability that a particular string will participate in the process of creating the new generation is proportional to a non-negative string performance index, called the string fitness, F(A).

High-fitness individuals will have a higher expected number of offsprings. Therefore, fitness proportionate reproduction guides the search towards the most promising direction. The steps described above are repeated for successive generations of the population, until an acceptable solution is found or until a fixed number of generations have evolved. The members in this generation with the highest level of fitness is the optical designs. The genetic operators crossover and mutation alter the structure of the strings to generate new offsprings for the next generation. This is illustrated later in the context of molecular design.

There is a large body of both theoretical and empirical evidence showing that even for very large an complex search spaces, genetic algorithms can rapidly locate structures with high fitness ratings (9, 14). However, to date, there exists no theoretical basis or proof guaranteeing convergence to global optimum. For more discussion on genetic algorithm fundamentals and applications the reader is referred to Holland.

Proposed Genetic Algorithm Framework for CAMD

In our proposed CAMD approach, for the forward problem, we use the standard group contribution methods which will be discussed later in the section on case studies. For the backward problem, we use the genetic algorithm which is presented in this section.

The standard genetic algorithm framework needs to be adapted for the molecular design problem. The modifications we introduced are in the string representation of molecules, creation of new operators that facilitate the chemistry of molecular interaction and rearrangements, and fitness function to handle property constraints. Figure 7.3 shows the proposed overall genetic algorithm framework for CAMD.

Molecule Representation

Bit string encoding is the most common coding scheme used by genetic algorithm researchers. Representing molecular structure as bit strings will result in binary matrices for representing the groups present in the structure and the connectivity among the groups. This representation makes the overall scheme more complicated because of the extensive book keeping needed and also makes the representation difficult to follow and interpret. Conceptually, a more suitable representation is to represent chemical structure as a string of symbols, as used by chemists. The string may be composed of one or more segments, each of which represents an elemental, substructural or monomer unit. Figure 7.3 presents examples of the symbolic coding scheme used in the present work, representing molecular structure as nested lists in Lisp (49). For the example in Figure 7.3, ((C C) I ((H H) (H Cl))), the first list of two Cs stand for two carbon backbone units. The subsequent lists contain elements that are sidechain substituents for each backbone unit in the order of the lists.

Adapting the Genetic Operators

In order to represent the richness and variety of the chemistry of molecular evolution, we had to develop new genetic operators (in addition to the crossover and mutation operators) not found in the standard genetic algorithm literature. The following describes the genetic operators used in this study.

One-Point Crossover

Figure 7.5 illustrates the one-point crossover operator. In this example, crossover occurs after position three of parent # 1 and position two of parent # 2 (as shown by the doted lines).

Blending Operator

The blending operator, produces one offspring from the end-to-end connection of two parents. This essentially combines the attributes from both parents. The molecular length is increased by applying the blending operator.

Mainchain Mutation and Sidechain Mutation

Mainchain and sidechain mutations are analogous to bit mutations. Mainchain and sidechain mutations are applied to the molecule as each groups along the main or sidechains are replaced by a randomly selected group.

Insertion and Deletion Operators

The insertion operator randomly inserts a group at a single mainchain or sidechain location. Similarly, the deletion operator randomly removes a small number of mainchain or sidechain groups. Removal of a sidechain group is equivalent to replacing the group with a hydrogen in the present work.

Hop Operator

When the hop operator is applied, a randomly selected group in the mainchain of the molecule 'hops to a randomly selected location on the mainchain. This facilitates small rearrangements in the ordering of the groups in a molecule, this causing a local search for the appropriate isomeric form that increases the fitness.

Genetic Search and Reproductive Plan

In genetic search, one needs to define a "goodness" function that is to be optimized over the evolution of several generations of candidates. This is a kind of score keeping, where the function scores the fitness or the merit of the candidate molecule. The candidate's fitness determines the probability of its participation in the evolution. In this study, two kinds of fitness functions are used depending on the nature of property constraints. When one is designing for a target property value with some bound (*i.e.* both upper and lower bounds on the desired value).

When the design involves property constraints that have only a lower bound or an upper bound, but not both.

Case Studies in Polymer Design

A common design problem in polymer engineering is to determine a polymer structure that can meet a number of physical properties constraints. We explored three case studies in this context. The first one is based on the design cases that had been investigated by Joback and Stephanopoulos (1989) (22), using their heuristic-guided enumeration approach. In their study, they had looked at cases for which the property constraints had a lower bound or an upper bound, but not both. The design problem gets to be more difficult if one were to consider constraints that are bounded both ways, particularly when the tolerance is tight. Venkatasubramanian (1996)(50), investigated this situation in case studies 2 and 3.

Case Study 1

In this case study, we demonstrate the performance of the genetic search framework for the polymers considered by Joback (1989)(21). Joback designed polymers that were required to satisfy the following property constraints.

1 Glass Transition Temperature Tg > 400 K

1 Volume Resistivity R > 1 × 1017 ohm-cm

1 Thermal Conductivity L > 1.6×10^7

1 Permeability to Oxygen P (O^2) < 1.0 cc-mil/100in 2/day/atm

Notice that these constraints have only one bound, lower or upper, but not both. Such constraints are easier to design for than those with both bounds and higher tolerances. Appropriate values for the genetic algorithm parameters such as the population size, operator probabilities, etc. are important for an efficient search. The various parameter values used in the case studies are shown in Table 7.2. A population of 100 members was used. Steady state reproduction was also used whereby the population remain fixed at all times. If no increasingly fit individual was discovered between generations, Venkatasubramanian (1996)(50) used the elitist policy by Grefenstette, 1986 (15), Goldberg, 1989 (14) of passing on ten of the most fit members of the population from the previous generation to the next. As one can see from Table 7.2, there are a number of parameters that can have a major impact on the design outcome. Choosing a suboptimal set of parameters can cause failure to discover the solution. This is a concern with the proposed approach. However, the literature contains more help on this matter in the form of rules of thumb for selecting the values of some of these parameters. A thorough parameter sensitivity and robustness analysis is required to understand these issues better. In that work, Venkarasubramanian (1996)(50), chose the parameter values after some limited experimentation. The values in Table 7.2, Joback reports that there are about 18,000 feasible molecules for this set of constraints and he lists fifty of them in his thesis (Joback, 1989)(21). The results of our genetic design framework are summarised in Table 7.3. For each independent run, Venkatasubramanian (1996)(50), allowed the genetic algorithm to evolve upto 100 generations, with a steady state population of 100 molecules. The table shows the number of distinct polymers found as well as the total number of molecules. The total number typically includes several copies of the same polymer. As one can observe, each run was successful and identified hundreds of solutions. The first solution was often found within the first 5-10 generations. When Venkatasubramanian (1996)(50), let the runs evolve for more generations (say, 500 or so), they found many more solutions. Since the constraints are open-ended and not tight, this is a relatively easier design problem and the genetic search is able to discover the desired polymers quite easily and quickly. One would expect the design problem to become more difficult if they tighten up the constraints. This is what they explored in case studies 2 & 3.

TABLE 7.1: Results for Case Study 1
Initial Population = 100, Total Generations = 100

Run #	*No. Distinct Solutions Found*	*Total No. Solutions Found*
1	1042	5278
2	1063	5274
3	1058	5204
4	1099	5434
5	1058	5161
6	1083	5530
7	1040	5215
8	999	5381
9	1032	5124
10	1049	5118
Average	1052.30	5271.90

TABLE 7.2: Results for Random Groups in Backbone and Sidechain Monomer Length 2 to 7

Target Polymer	*Average Generation No. when First Solution was Found*	*Average No. of Solutions at the End of GA Search*
Poly (vinylidene propylene) copolymer	11.3	14.0
Polythylene terephthalate	28.2	10.5
Polycabonate of bisphenol-A	41.0	3.9

TABLE 7.3: Results for Random –CH2– Groups Monoluer Length 2 to 7

Target Polymer	*Average Generation No. when First Solution was Found*	*Average No. of Solutions at the End of GA Search*
Poly (vinylidene propylene) copolymer	11.3	14.3
Polythylene terephthalate	13.6	11.3
Polycabonate of bisphenol-A	58.8	3.8

Case Study 2

In this case study, Venkatasubramanian (1996)(50), introduced the following features to make the design problem more complex than the first case study. First, they allowed for independent changes of the groups in the side chain as well as in the backbone of the polymers. In case study 1, the sidechain groups could not be changed independently. Next they tightened up the constraints. Here, the task was to design a molecule whose property values were within ±0.5 per cent of the target properties. It is important to note here that this tolerance is very tight and makes the search more difficult. Previous efforts in molecular design had not considered such tight constraints. Finally, they increased the number of constraints from four to five. The property constraints that were considered in this case study were density, glass transition temperature, linear thermal expansion coefficient, dielectric constant, and specific heat capacity. The properties were calculated by using van Krevelen's group contribution methods proposed by van Krevelen and Hoftyzer, 1976 (43).

In this study, the mainchain and sidechain base groups were chosen such that the group contribution parameters were available for all the properties considered and that the molecules constructed by the genetic operators satisfied normal chemical bonding constraints. Chemically infeasible group combinations could be avoided by represent complex chemical interaction and arrangement constraints with relative case is one of the appeals of the proposed approach. To examine the ability of the genetic algorithm framework for polymer design, Venkatasubramanian (1996)(50), chose three target polymers that offer different levels of difficulty in design. They are: (i) Polyethylene terephthalate (PET), (ii) Polyvinylidene propylene copolymer (PVP), and (iii) Polycarbonate of bisphenol-A (PC). PET is the simplest and the polycarbonate is the most difficult of the three. This is so because PC has non-linear group interactions where the ordering of the groups matter in determining the properties and hence the search space is more complex. The properties of these target molecules were computed using the group contribution methods of van Krevelen and Hoftyzer, (1976) (43) and are listed in Table 7.5. These were submitted, one molecule at a time, to the genetic algorithm based CAMD system as the target properties with a tolerance of ±0.5 per cent in the property values.

TABLE 7.4: Results for Random Groups and Sidechain Monomer Length 2 to 10

Target Polymer	*Average Generation Number when First Solution was Found*	*Average Number of Monomers Found at the End of GA Search*	*Average Number of Dimers Found at the end of GA Search*
Poly (vinylidene propylene) copolymer	12.1	6.7	14.8
Polythylene terephthalate	28.4	9.1	7.8
Polycabonate of bisphenol-A	60.6	2.9	5.8

TABLE 7.5: Results for Random –CH2– Groups Monomer Length 2 to 10

Target Polymer	*Average Generation Number when First Solution was Found*	*Average Number of Monomers Found at the End of GA Search*	*Average Number of Dimers Found at the end of GA Search*
Poly (vinylidene propylene) copolymer	12.4	6.9	13.9
Polythylene terephthalate	14.7	8.5	8.1
Polycabonate of bisphenol-A	73.1	1.7	3.5

Polymer Design Case Studies

As one can see from the success rate, the genetic search did very well in general. For the polymers PET and PVP, the search discovered these polymers in every run. Furthermore, it discovered multiple instances of these polymers with exactly the same structure and also found them fairly quickly as seen from the low average generation count. In addition, it also found several other structures which had very high fitness values (typically, 0.90 or better). It took longer to find the solution for L=10 in comparison with L=7, as the search space is larger for the former. It is interesting to note that for L=10 case, the genetic search discovered dimers as well as monomers. With respect to computational effort, the longest run took about 5 minutes in real-time (about 2 cpu secs) on a Sparc 10 workstation. Our genetic algorithm program has not been optimized and there is considerable room for significant improvements in speed.

The Polycarbonate is the most difficult as mentioned before. Hence, on an average, it took more generations to discover this polymer. The genetic search discovered this polymer with 100 per cent success rate for L=7 case. For the L=10 case, it was less successful (76 per cent) when the initial population was a random collection of —CH2- chains. This is so because the members of the initial population were very different in their structure from the target and hence it took longer to discover the correct groups and structure. Venkatasubramanian (1996) (50), observed that if they let the able to discover the target in most cases. In the case of random groups initialization, some of the right groups (like benzene or OCO) were already be present in the starter population. This gave a better start and hence a quicker search.

Case Study 3

In this case study, Venkatasubramanian (1996) (50), revisited Joback's cases with tighter constraints. They identified ten polymers of different lengths and complexity from Joback's list (1989) (21), and chose their properties as the target to design for. This time, however, the constraints were tightened. The task was to design a molecule whose property values were within ±0.5 per cent of the target properties. If the genetic search were to be successful, it should discover all the ten molecules, one at a time. Researchers used the same genetic search parameters as shown in Table 7.2 with a gaussian fitness function. Each target polymer was attempted ten times, in ten different runs. In each run, the starting population consisted of random polymers made of groups in Table 7.1. In each run, the population was allowed to evolve upto 500 generations. Values such as generation count and number of solutions are always integer values in individual runs, but the result summarizes averages over 10 runs and hence they have real values. As one can see from the success rate, the genetic search did quite well in general. All the ten molecules were discovered by the genetic search, though some more often and quickly than others. For example, molecule # 10 was found fairly quickly (in about 40 generations on an average) and also was found in every run, (thus, a success rate of 100 per cent). On the other hand, some other polymer like # 9 took much longer (about 315 generations on an average) and also with a smaller success rate (3 of the 10 runs were unsuccessful in discovering this polymer). Typically, a molecule that is longer and has more diversity of groups in its structure takes longer to discover. Other factors such as how close the alternate solutions are to the target molecule also matter considerably as the genetic search could get stuck in such local optima.

Whenever the genetic search failed to discover the target polymer, it always came up with several solution structures that had very high fitness (typically 0.95 or higher). Many of these alternatives were structurally quite similar to the target. It is important to note that this ability of the genetic design framework to provide a collection of possible alternatives that are of high fitness is a very useful design feature.

Random Search for Molecular Design

The performance of any molecular design algorithm is dependent upon a number of factors such as the physical property constraints, estimation procedures, base group set, allowable range of group repetitions, algorithm parameters and so on. However, it is instructive to identify a baseline of comparison for CAMD methodologies by examining the corresponding combinatorial complexity associated with exhaustive enumeration and the success rate of a random search. If one assumes that the changes in group ordering do not affect physical properties (as is the case with most instances of the group contribution methods).

For example, designs of length 1-7 using 7 backbone and sidechain groups yield 88 million possible design candidates.

For the purposes of comparison, Venkatasubramanian (1996) (50), implemented a random search technique on Joback's polymer design case study with close-ended design constraints. Analogous to the genetic algorithm case study, 100 polymers per generation were generated for 500 generations for a total of 50,000 design candidates in a single run. This was repeated for 10 runs for each design study. The random search procedure consisted of randomly selecting a length of 1 through 7 groups and then randomly filling in the mainchain elements with groups from Table 7.1. The results from such a random search is compared with that of the genetic search. As one would expect, the random search did rather well for smaller molecules (*i.e.* with 4 base groups) as the number of possibilities are not very large. However, the random search performs poorly for larger molecules where the possibilities become combinatorially large. This is where the advantage of using the genetic search becomes more apparent.

Survival by Fitness

With the proper equations, data can be tested to determine the best-performing member of any set. Then, as in nature, the fittest remain and weak become extinct. According to Globis (12), "The key to any genetic software solution is a good fitness function. This function must be very robust since the randomly generated initial molecules rarely make chemical sense". The first step, however, is to convert the genetic representation of the molecules into the molecular structure, similar to the way proteins are made based on DNA and RNA. Once the molecules are built, the fitness function is applied. For drug discovery, the fitness function is the same as ranks the molecules; the poorest docking compounds are removed; and the remainder are modified genetically.

Fitness functions are extremely complex and tax the computer that run them. Typically, the functions must not only build the molecules, but also calculate the properties based on what was learned in the first structure-to-properties stage. Then they determine the effect when the molecule with properties attached is placed on the receptor. This is further complicated by the fact that in the three-dimensional world, there are many ways the drug molecule could approach the receptor. Some more recent programs allow for flexibility and even the presence of water between the receptor and the molecule. Unfortunately, these enhancements often take even more computing power. In essence, the entire process is limited by the speed of the fitness function.

Companies Using Genetic Algorithms

Currently, most major pharmaceutical companies use rational drug design and evolutionary techniques such as genetic algorithms as part of the drug discovery process. Several small pharma companies have also made innovations in this area. Companies such as Tripos, Daylight Chemical Information Systems, Axys Pharmaceuticals, and Nanodesign, among others, market products and services to small and large pharmaceutical and biotech companies that are based on genetic algorithms. Tripos has developed several software products and services using genetic algorithms. Within its SYBYL program, the company offers a genetic algorithm- based conformational search tool for exploring the three-dimensional shapes that molecules attain. The GASP algorithm measures similarity and overlays molecules based on matches between their hydrogen bond donors / acceptors, hydrophobes, etc. The company has also been using genetic algorithms on binding problems. Flexidock uses a genetic algorithm to fit ligands into protein binding sites and accounts for conformational flexibility. Tripos is also working with collaborators to develop new tools, such as a de nove ligand design toolkit based on evolutionary principles under development at the University of Texas-Austin.

Daylight Chemical Information Systems, Inc., owns a 1993 patent on an evolutionary technique that uses SMILES strings as genetic material and performs fitness functions using comparative molecular field analysis (CoMFA), (SMILES, or simplified linear form). Axys Pharmaceuticals also has a patent describing a neural network-based approach to modelling activity and designing new compounds.

Nanodesign has developed technology to provide novel chemical structure as candidates for the pharmaceutical industry. It uses a computational drug design process called Evolutionary Molecular Design (EMD). This process identifies the activity that is required for the receptor and focuses on the ligand structure rather than the receptor structure. Once the required activity has been identified for the receptor, a molecular assembler is used to identify structures that meet the requirements identified for the receptor. The most interesting facet of Nanodesign's approach is the use of genetic algorithms to generate both the virtual receptor and the new ligands. Therefore, Nanodesign's EMD uses genetic algorithms in both the forward and reverse probe. Obviously, these companies are striving for new drug developments by using computational methods that achieve greater accuracy than could previously be obtained using older drug development tools.

Conclusions

The feasibility of utilizing a genetic algorithm framework for computer-assisted molecular design has been demonstrated with examples in polymer design. This study opens up a new avenue of possibilities in rational approaches to molecular design that could have a significant impact on a wide variety or molecular design problems. As mentioned in the Introduction, present CAMD approaches such as exhaustive enumeration and heuristics-guided enumeration suffer from the problem of combinatorial complexity of dealing with millions of possible candidates for large, complex molecules. In the knowledge-based approach, acquisition of the appropriate heuristics is a serious problem. While the MINLP formalism has a certain appeal due to its rigorous mathematical foundation, it suffers from local minima traps. In addition, in many practical design situations it may be extremely difficult or even impossible to express the non-linear structure-property correlations within the MINLP framework.

In contrast, the proposed genetic algorithm framework offers a number of advantages, such as—it is a multiple point search technique that examines a set of solutions and not just one solution—this and the stochastic nature of the algorithm helps the search to escape local minima traps; it is not derivative-based, thus avoiding the difficulties faced by math programming techniques in this respect; it is relatively easy to express the rich and complex chemistry of molecules; one can integrate whatever heuristic knowledge one might have about the problem quite easily into the genetic framework to speed up the design process. For instance, instead of starting the initial population at random, the designer can start with structures that are good guesses based on his or her experience; it provides a set of alternate solutions and not just one. This would be particularly useful for the design of complex molecules where the forward problem results may not be completely reliable. Hence one would like a collection of design candidates that are fairly close to each other to test further with actual synthesis and experimentation in a laboratory.

On the down side, the proposed approach suffers from two main drawbacks. One is the heuristic nature of the search and that is no guarantee of finding the best solution. But then, this criticism would be applicable to the other heuristic approaches mentioned above as well. Even in the MINLP approach, there is no guarantee of a global optimum solution. The other drawback is the selection of the parameter values which would requires some experimentation.

Simulated annealing may have some appeal for the molecular design problem, but it has not been tried yet. But the standard simulated annealing needs to be modified in order to express the rich chemistry of this problem domain, by introducing the equivalent of the various genetic operators. If one were to make the appropriate changes and also introduce the multiple-point search (which is not present in the standard simulated annealing approach), one would have developed a technique that is essentially like the genetic algorithm.

The key advantage of genetic algorithms is that they not only use the computer as a tool for modelling and understanding properties, but also enable the computer to develop new structures and determine whether those structures serve a specific purpose. This allows discoveries of a random, almost accidental nature. Accidents made by humans have led to some of the greatest scientific discoveries of all time. Venkatasubramanian concluded that one of the advantages (of evolutionary techniques) was not so much that it may have produced an explicit structure which -was an immediate winner, but it forced them (the researchers) to think outside the box. Although Venkatasubramanian was discussing engineering materials in this case, the same could be true of pharmaceuticals. Genetic algorithms show the potential for researchers. This advantage may increase the yield of discovery, dramatically influencing the development of pharmaceuticals in the coming decades.

Acknowledgement

In the preparation of this chapter, help has been taken from various source material which has been duly acknowledge. We are also grateful to V. Venkatasubramanian, K. Chan and J.M. Caruthers of Purdue University, USA for their kind help.

References

1. Aoyama, A. and Ventakatasubramanian, V. (1995). Internal Model Control Framework Using Neural Networks for the Modelling and Control of a Bioreactor. *Engg. Applic. Artif. Intell.,* In press.
2. Aoyama, T., Suzuki, Y., and Ichikawa, H. (1990). Neural Networks Applied to Quantitative Structure-activity Relationship. *J. Med. Chem.,* 33(3): 905-908.
3. Androulakis, I.P. and V. Venkatasubramanian (1991). A Genetic Algorithm Framework for Process Design and Optimization. *Computer Chem. Engg.,* 15(4): 217-228.
4. Bolis, G., Pace, L.D. and Fabrocini, F. (1991). A Machine Learning Approach to Computer-aided Molecular Design. *Journal of Computer-aided Molecular Design,* 5: 617-628.
5. Brignole. E.A., Bottlini, S. and Gani, R. (1986). A Strategy for Design and Selection of Solvents for Separation Processes. *Fluid Phase Equilibria,* 29: 125.
6. Burkert, U. and Allinger. N.L. (1982). *Molecular Mechanics.* ACS Monogram 177, American Chemical Society, Washington, DC.
7. Cybenko, G. (1988). Approximation by Superpositions of Sigmoidal Functions. *Math. of Cont. Syst. Sig.,* 2: 303-314.
8. Derringer, G.C. and Markham, R.L. (1985). A Computer-based Methodology for Matching Polymer Structure with Required Properties. *Journal of Applied Polymer Science,* 30: 4609-4617.
9. Davis, D. (ed) (1991). *Handbook of Genetic Algorithms.* Van Nostrand Reinhold.
10. Elrod, D. W., Maggiora, G.M. and Trenary, R.G. (1990). Applications of Neural Networks in Chemistry I: Prediction of Electrophilic Aromatic Substitution Reactions. *Chem. Inf Comput. Sci.,* 30(4): 477-484.

11. Gani, R., and Brignole, E.A. (1983). Molecular Design of Solvents for Liquid Extraction Based on UNIFAC. *Fluid Phase Equilibria,* 13: 331-340.

12. Globis, A. (1999). Automatic Molecular Design Using Evolutionary Techniques. *Nanotechnology,* 10(3): 290-299.

13. Gani, R., Nielsen, B. and Fredenslund, A. (1991). A Group Contribution Approach to Computer-aided Molecular Design. *AIChE Journal,* 37(9): 1318-1332.

14. Goldberg, D.E. (1989). *Genetic Algorithm in Search, Optimization, and Machine Learning*. Addisson-Wesley.

15. Grefenstette, J.J. (1986). Optimization of Control Parameters for Genetic Algorithms. IEEE *Transactions of System, Man and Cybernetics,* 16: 122-128.

16. Holland, J.H. (1975). *Adaptation in Natural and Artificial Systems.* University of Michigan Press, Ann Arbor.

17. Hibbet, D.B. (1993). Genetic Algorithm in Chemistry. *Chemometrics and Intelligent Laboratory Systems,* 19: 277-293.

18. Holland, J.H. (1975). *Adaptation in Natural and Artificial System.* The University of Michigan Press. Ann Arbor.

19. Hopfinger, A.J., Koehler, M.G. and Pearlstein, R.A. (1988). Molecular Modelling of Polymers, IV. Estimation of Glass Transition Temperatures. *J. Polym. Sci., Part B: Polym. Phys.,* 26: 2007-2028.

20. Joback, K.G. and Reid, R.C. (1987). Estimation of Pure-component Properties from Group Contributions, *Chem. Eng. Comm.,* 57: 233-243.

21. Joback, K.G. (1989). *Design Molecular Possessing Desired Physical Property Values, Volume 1 and* 2. Ph. D. Thesis 10 Chemical Engineering, MIT.

22. Joback, K.G. and Stephanopoulos, G. (1989). Designing Molecules Possessing Desired Physical Property Values. In: *Proceedings of FOCAPD'89,* Snowmass, Co., 363-387.

23. Jurs, P.C. and Isenhour, T.L. (1975). *Chemical Applications of Pattern Recognition.* Wiley and Sons, New York.

24. Joback, K.G. (1989). Designing Molecules Possessing Desired Physical Property Values, Ph. D. Thesis, M.I.T., Cambridge, MA.

25. Kier, L.B. and Hall, L.H. (1986). *Molecular Connectivity in Structure-activity Analysis*, Research Studies Press, Letchworth, Hertfordshire, U.K.

26. Kier, L.B. and Hall, L.H. (1976). *Molecular Connectivity in Chemistry and Drug Research.* Academic Press, New York.

27. Kier, L.B., Lowell, H.H. and Frazer, J.F. (1993). Design of Molecules from Quantitative Structure-activity Relationship Models. I. Information Transfer Between Path and Vertex Degree Counts. *J. Chem. Inf. Comput. Sci.*, 33.

28. Koehler, M.G., and Hopfinger, A.J. (1989). Molecular Modelling of Polymers: 5. Inclusion of Intermolecular Energetics in Estimating Glass and Crystal-Melt Tansition Temperatures. *Polymer*, 30: 116-126.

29. Macchietto, S., Odele, O. and Omatsome, O. (1990). Design of Optimal Solvents for Liquid-Liquid Extraction and Gas Absorption Processes. *Trans. Ind. ChemE.*, 68A: 429-433.

30. Nagasaka, K., H. Wada, H. Yoshimitsu, H. Yasuda, and T. Yamanouchi (1990). Expert system for Polymer Design. *41ChE Annual Meeting*, 39E, Chicago, IL, November.

31. Orchard, B.J., Tripathy, S.K., Pearlstein, R.A., and Hopfinger, A.J. (1987). Molecular Modelling of Polymer: I. Corrected and Efficient Enumeration of the Intrachain Conformational Energetics. *J. Comput. Chem.*, 8(1): 28-38.

32. Psichogios, D.C. and Ungar, L.H. (1992). A Hybrid Neural Network-first Principles Approach to Process Modelling. *AIChE Journal.*, 38: 1499-1512.

33. Qian, N. and Sejnowski, T.J. (1988). Predicting the Secondary Structure of Globular Proteins using Neural Network Models. *J. Mol. Biol.*, 202: 865-884.

34. Reid, R.C., Prausnitz, J.M. and Sherwood, T.K. (1977). *The Properties of Gases and Liquids.* McGraw-Hill, New York.

35. Reid, R.C., Prausnitz, J.M. and Poling, B.E., (1987). *The Properties of Gases and Liquids.* McGraw-Hill, New York.

36. Rose, V.S., Macfie, H.J.H. and Croall, I.F. (1991). *Pharmacochem. Libr.*, 16: 213-216.

37. Robb, H.W. and Munk, M.H. (1990). A Neural Network Approach to Infrared Spectrum Interpretation. *Mikrochim Acta*, 31-155.

38. Skvortsova, M.I., Baskin, I.I.., Slovokhotova, O.L., Palyulin, V.A., and Zefirov, N.S. (1993). Inverse Problem in QSAR/QSPR Studies for the Case of Topological Indices Characterizing Molecular Shape (Kier Indices). *J. Chem. Inf. Comput. Sci.*, 33(4): 630-634.

39. Sumpter, B.G., Gettino, C., Noid, D.W. (1994). Theory and Applications of Neural Computing in Chemical Science. *Annu. Rev. Phys. Chem.*, 45: 439-481.

40. Sumpter, B.G. and Noid, D.W. (1994). *Makromol. Chem. Theory Simul.*, 3: 363-378.

41. Strouf, O. (1986). *Chemical Pattern Recognition*. Research Studies Press.

42. Van Krevelen, D.W. and Hoftyzer, P.J. (1972). *Properties of Polymers, their Estimation and Correlation with Chemical Structure*, First Edition. Elsevier Scientific.

43. Van Krevelen, D.W. and Hoftyzer, P.I. (1976). *Properties of Polymers, their Estimation and Correlation with Chemical Structure*, Second Edition. Elsevier Scientific.

44. Van Krevelen, D.W., and Hoftyzer, P.I. (1990). *Properties of Polymers, their Estimation and Correlation with Chemical Structure*, Third Edition. Elsevier Scientific.

45. Venkatasubramanian, V., Chan, K. and Caruthers, J.M. (1994). Computer-aided Molecular Design Using Genetic Algorithms. *Computers Chem. Engg.*, 18(9): 833-844.

46. Venkatasubramanian, V., Chan, K. and Carutherst J.M. (1995). Evolutionary Design of Molecules with Desired Properties using the Genetic Algorithm. *J. Chem. Comput: Sci.*, 35: 188-195.

47. Wythoff, B.I., Levine, S.P., and Tomellinit S.A. (1990). *Anal. Chem.*, 62: 2702-2709.

48. Zupan, J. and Gasteiger, J. (1991). *Neural Networks: A New Method for Solving Chemical Problems or Just a Passing Phase?* Technical

Report, TU Munchen, D-8046, Garching, Organisch-Chemisches Institute Germany.

49. Winston, P.H. and Horn, B.K.P. (1985). *LISP*, Second Edition, Addison-Wesley Publishing Co., Reading, MA.

50. Venkatsubramanian, V., (1996). Computer-aided Molecular Design Using Neural Networks and Genetic Algorithms. In: *Genetic Algorithms in Molecular Modelling;* Delivers, J. (Ed.), Academic Press, New York.

51. Venkatasubramanian, V., Chan, K. and Curuthers, J.M. (1992). Designing Engineering Polymers: A Case Study in Product Design, *AIChE Annual Meeting*, 140d, Maimi, FL, November.

CHAPTER 8

Genomic Image Processing and Analysis for Development of New Genomic Medicine

Introduction

Genomic image processing and analysis is most important for visualizing and critical analysis of the genome from microarray and 2-D Gel Electrophoresis of Genomic DNA so that new genomic drug can be developed. This chapter describes the images types and their algorithm, the preocess and the steps of image analysis through target segmentation, background intensity extraction, target detection, target intensity extraction, ratio analysis, multiple image analysis, lastly analysis through software package.

Images are the arrays of pixels. The values of the image's pixels arc stored in disk files and when an image is displayed in a picture box or from control, each one of its pixels is mapped to a pixels on the picture box or from. In this point of view, image processing is nothing more than simple arithmetic operation on the values of the image pixels.

The objective of the Genomic image processing is needed mainly for-microarray analysis to extract probe intensities or ratios at each cDNA target location, and then cross-link printed clone target information so that biologists can easily interpret the outcomes and perform further high-level analysis (1) and Image Processing for 2-D Gel Electrophoresis of Genomic DNA.

However, the microarray image sources are not only from one print-mode (*i.e.*, number of printing tips) or one hybridization method (*i.e.*, fluorescent or radioactive probe). Nevertheless, in order to simplify the presentation of information for this section we have chosen to model the microarray images below from *two fluorescent probes* are our main processing input images.

How the Image Application Works?

At first the image is loaded on a picture box control. Now the values of its pixels are accessed with the point method, which returns a long integer representing each pixel color. The basic color components must be extracted from long value used to implement the algorithms (7).

This is a time consuming step, and for most algorithms, it must be performed more than once for each pixels. To speed up the processing, one can choose to read the values of all the pixels when the image is loaded and store them in an array (2).

The array stored the values of the pixels called *'Image-pixels'* with visual basic is declared as follows:

Global Imagepixels (2,800,800) as Integer

There are tow for reading the image pixels into image pixels array-using the point method or read the pixels directly from the file.

The point method is simpler which reads the pixel values directly off the picture box. But most image processing application use the other options, reading the pixels directly from the file. This technique is faster and have to supply image type (Visual Basic supports three Image type: BMP, GIP and JPEG). In this process, the program calls the open command dialog box, which lets the user select an image and then loads the image on the picture-box.

The picture-box's 'Scale-mode' property is set to 3 (pixels) and it's 'Auto-size' is set to true. Image dimensions can find out from picture box dimensions. If the image dimensions exceeds 800, the process ends with appropriate message and the image does not loaded. If the image's dimensions are smaller, the program proceeds by reading the pixels values into the *'Image-pixels'* array. The value returned by the point method in long integer, which contents all three color-components (Red, Green, Blue). Three color component extract with the Get Red (R), Get Green (G) and Get Blue (B) functions. Once extracted, the color components are stored in the appropriate elements of the *'Image-pixel'* array. The first index in the array corresponds to a color component (0 for red, 1 for green, 2 for blue), the second index to the pixels column, the third index to the pixels row.

The code behind the open command in Visual Basic 0.6 is following:

```
Private Sub File Open_Click(–)
Dim i As Integer, j As Integer
Dim red as Integer, Dim green as Integer, Dim blue as Integer
Dim pixel as long
Dim Picture name as String
ComonDialog1.IntDir = App.Path
CommonDialog1.Filter – "Images| *.BMP;*.GIF;*.JPJ;*.DIB| All Files| *.*"
ComonDialog1.Actlon = 1
PictureName = CommonDialog1.File Name
**If Picture Name = " " Then Exit Sub
Picture1.Picture = LoadPicture (PictureName)
Form1.Refresh
X = Picture1.ScleWidth
Y = Picture1.ScleHeight
If X > 500 or Y > 500 then
MsgBox "Image too large to process. Please try loading a smaller
   image"
X = 0
Y = 0
Exit Sub
Exit If
From1.Width = Form1.ScaleX(Picture1.Width + 6, vbPixels, vbTwips)
From1.Height = Form1.ScaleY(Picture.Height + 30, vbPixels, vbTwips)
From1.Refresh
From3.Show
From3.Refresh
For i = 0 to Y-1
For j = 0 to X-1
Pixel = Form1.Picture1.Point(j,i)
red = pixel and  Mod 256
green = (pixel And  &Hff00)/256&) Mod 256&
```

```
blue = (pixel and &Hff000)/65536
ImagePixels (0,I,J) = red
ImagePixels (1,I,j) = green
ImagePixels (2,I,j) = blue
Next
From3.Progressbar1. Value = I* 100/(y-l)
Next
Form3.Hide
End Sub
```

Using the image applications One can apply the effects to an image any one of the detail), *Emboss* (add a raised look), *Diffuse* (gives a painterly look, *Solarize* (creates a special effect based on selective pixels inversion) (2, 3, 8). The algorithm of different types of images arc following:

The Smooth Image Algorithm

To smooth a image, one must reduces the large difference adjustment of pixels. In time of calculation, nine pixels are assume and it also assume that all the pixels in this block is green except middle one, which is red. This pixels drastically different from it's neighbors, for it to be blurred, it must be pulled towards the average of the other pixels. Taking the average of a block of pixels is, therefore, a good choice blurring operation.

The Smooth Image Algorithm in Visual Basic 0.6 is following:

```
Private Sub ProcessSmooth_Click(–)
Dim i As Integer, j As Integer
Dim red as Integer, Dim green as Integer, Dim blue as Integer
For i = 1 to Y-2
For j = 1 to X -2
Red = ImagePixels (0, i-1, j-1)
+ ImagePixels (0, i-1, j) + ImagePixels (0, i-1, j+1)_
+ ImagePixels (0, i, j-1) + ImagePixels (0, i, j)_
+ ImagePixels (0, i, j+1) + ImagePixels (0, i+1, j-1)_
+ ImagePixels (0, i+1, j) + ImagePixels (0, i+1, j+1)
green = ImagePixels (1, i-1, j-1)_
+ ImagePixels (1, i-1, j) + ImagePixels (1, i-1, j+1)_
+ ImagePixels (1, i, j-1) + ImagePixels (1, i, j)_
+ ImagePixels (1, i, j+1) + ImagePixels (1, I+1, j-1)_
+ ImagePixels (1, i+1, j) + ImagePixels (1, i+1, j+1)
blue = ImagePixels (2, i-1, j-1)_
+ ImagePixels (2, i-1, j) + ImagePixels (2, i-1, j+1)_
```

```
+ ImagePixels (2, i, j-1) + ImagePixels (2, i, j)_
+ ImagePixels (2, i, j+1) + ImagePixels (2, i+1, j-1)_
+ ImagePixels (2, i+1, j) + ImagePixels (2, I+1, j+1)
picture1.Pset (j, i), RGB (red/9, green/9, blue/9)
Next
Picture1.Referesh
Next
End Sub
```

The Sharpen Image Algorithm

In a sharpen image the different between two adjacent pixels will be large value (may be negative) but in smooth image different between two adjacent pixels will be zero or a very small. The question is now how to bring out the detail without levelling the rest of the image and how about adding to the original pixel? Where the image is flat, the difference is negligible, and the processed pixel practically will be the same as original one.

The Sharpen Image Algorithm in Visual Basic 0.6 (new_value = original_value + 0.5 * difference) is following:

```
Private Sub ProcessSharpen_Click(–)
Dim i As Integer, j As Integer
Dim Dx As Integer = 1
Dim Dy As Integer = 1
Dim red as Integer, Dim green as Integer, Dim blue as Integer
For i= 1 to Y-2
For j = 1 to X-2
red = ImagePixels (0, i, j) + 0.5* ImagePixels (0, i, j)_
   – ImagePixels (0, i-Dx, j-Dy)
green = ImagePixels (1, i, j) + 0.5* ImagePixels (1, i, j)_
   – ImagePixels (1 i-Dx, j-Dy)
blue = ImagePixels (2, i, j) + 0.5* ImagePixels (2, i, j)
   – ImagePixels (2, i-Dx, j-Dy)
If red > 255 then red = 255
If red < 0 then red = 0
If green > 255 then green = 255
If green < 0 then green = 0
If blue > 255 then blue = 255
If blue < 0 then blue = 0
Picture1.Pset (j, i) RGB (red, green, blue)
Next
End Sub
```

The Emboss Image Algorithm

The emboss image looks as raised and illuminated. This effect is known as emboss or bas relief. The emboss algorithm adds a constant to the difference to bring some brightness to areas of the image that would otherwise be dark. The algorithm can be expressed as follows: new_value – difference 128

The code that implements the emboss filter in the image application uses differences in the X and y directions (set the values of the variables Dx or Dy to take the difference in none direction only).

The Emboss Filter Code in Visual Basic 0.6 is following:

```
Private Sub ProcessEmboss_Click(–)
Dim i As Integer, j As Integer
Dim Dx As Integer = 1
Dim Dy As Integer = 1
Dim red as Integer, Dim green as Integer, Dim blue as Integer
For i = 1 to Y –2
For j = 1 to X –2
Red = Abs(ImagePixels (0, 1, j)_
   –ImagePixels (0, i+Dx, j+Dy) + 128)
Green = Abs(ImagePixels (1, I, j)_
   –ImagePixels (1, i+Dx, j+Dy) + 128)
Blue = Abs(ImagePixels (2, I, j)_
   –ImagePixels ((2, I+Dx, j+Dy) + 128)
Picture1.Pset (j, i), RGB(red, green, blue)
Next
Picture1.Refresh
Next
End Sub
```

The Diffuse Image Algorithm

The diffuse image is not based on the sums or the difference of pixel values. The diffuse special effect uses the Rnd() function to introduce some randomness to the image and give it a painterly look.

The Diffuse Image Algorithm in Visual Basic 6.0 is following:

```
Private Sub ProcessDiffuse_Click(–)
Dim i As Integer, j As Integer
```

```
Dim Rx As Integer, Dim Ry As Integer = 1
Dim red as Integer, Dim green as Integer, Dim blue as Integer
For i = 2 to Y -3
For j = 2 to X -3
Rx = Rnd () *4 -2
Ry = Rnd () *4 -2
red = ImagePixels (0, i+Rx, j+Ry)
green = ImagePixels (1, i+Rx, j+Ry)
blue = ImagePixels (2, i+Rx, j+Ry)
picture1.Pset (j, i), RGB(red, green, blue)
Next
  DoEvents
Next
End Sub
```

The Solarize Image Algorithm

This effect in the image application is based on a photographic technique. This technique is called solarization. The alogrithm as implemented in the image application inverts the basic colour components whose values are less than 128.

The Solarize Image Algorithm in Visual Basic 0.6 is following:

```
Private Sub Process.Solarize_Click(–)
Dim i As Integer, j As Integer
Dim red as Integer, Dim green as Integer, Dim blue as Integer
For i = 1 to Y -2
For j = 1 to X -2
Red = ImagePixels (0, i, j)
Green = ImagePixels (1, i, j)
Blue = ImagePixels (2, i, j)
  Red = 225 -red
If ((green < 128) or (green > 225) then_
  Green = 225 -green
If ((blue < 128) or (blue > 225) then_
  Blue = 225 -blue
Picture1.Pset (i, j) RGB(red, green, blue)
Next
  DoEvents
Next
Picture1.Refresh
End Sub
```

Genomic Image Processing and Analysis

For this particular image example, an array of cDNAs was hyrbidized with a red flour-tagged sample and green flour-tagged sample, and then monochrome images of the fluorescent intensity were combined by placing each image into the appropriate colour channel of the RGB colour image. In this experiment, there were a total of 1,344 cDNA targets (printed from fourteen 96-well plates) using four print-tips, by defining the print-mode, the software can track the cDNA targets on this and the other array and map them back to their original plate position.

Image Processing and analysis can be divided into following tasks:

1. Target segmentation.
2. Background intensity extraction.
3. Target detection.
4. Target intensity extraction.
5. Ratio analysis.
6. Multiple image analysis.
7. Genome analysis software package.

Target Segmentation

Since each element of an array is printed automatically to a defined position, one can safely assume that the final probe signals form a regular array which can be automatically aligned to a predefined grid-overlay. The initial position of the grid, as shown in the picture, can be either (I) manually determined if no particular orientation markers (called "landing lights") are printed or no visible signals from the orientation markers (or II), automatically determined if the orientation markers are presented in the final image and the entire array has no obvious missing row or column signals. Due to the complication of the customized print procedures and various hybridization protocols, we assume the initial grid-overly is manually determined.

Usually, the initial overlay grid does not precisely segment the targets. The refinement of the grid position is preferably done automatically. The procedure we utilize is as follows: (1) detect strong targets, (2) find their centers (*e.g.*, center of mass), (3) regress four-corner coordinates of each sub-array from these centers of strong signals. This last regression step is important since it avoids the problem of false centers due to noise blobs or miscalculated centers. The final grid-overlay precisely segments each target, which enables future processing tasks to concentrate only one target. Also, the target position can be deconvoluted back to its original microplate position when the printing information is available on-line. Thus, the clone information can be attached to each target at this stage.

Background Intensity Extraction

The background of the microarray image is not uniform over the entire array and therefore it is necessary to extract local background intensity. The changes of fluorescent background across an array is usually gradual and smooth, and may be due to many technical reasons. Abrupt changes are rare, when they happen, the actual signal intensities of array elements near these changes are not reliable. Conventionally, pixels near the bounding box edge are taken to be background pixels, and thus the mean gray-level of these pixels provides an estimation of the local background intensity. This method become inaccurate when bonding box size is close to 10 × 10 pixels, or the target fills entire bounding box.

Fluorescent background is typically modelled by a Gaussian process. For example, if one choose a larger area (*e.g.*, a 30 × 30 box centered at a particular target) the gray-level histogram within the box is usually unimodal since the majority of the background pixel values are similar while the target pixel values spread up to vary high gray levels. The location of the mode of the histogram, therefore, provides the mean local background intensity and the left tail of the histogram will provide the spread (standard deviation) of the background intensity.

Target Detection

One of the difficult image processing tasks is to identify the target region within the bounding box. Each target is somewhat annular, resulting form both how the robot finger places the cDNA on the slide and how the slide is treated. However, the final image of the target may simply be a collection of subregions within the nominal circular target region due to the variability introduced by cDNA deposition or the hybridization process. It is important that the final signal intensity be measured over regions corresponding to probe-hybridized-to-target area.

Conventionally a fixed thresholding method is used in image analysis. The threshold value *T* can be determined form the local background mean intensity *m* and its standard deviations by the relationship '*T*' = *m* + 3 s. However, the simple fixed thresholding method fails quite often due to variability of the background and the signal, particularly when the signal is weak (a frequent finding in cDNA array experiments). To avoid these problems, some sophisticated thresholding methods may be implemented. One of the methods that we utilize is the Mann-Whitney method, which takes sample pixels form the background and then performs a rank-sum hypothesis test on the target pixels. This approach allows users to specify the confidence level of target detection.

Target Intensity Extraction

After target regions are determine, intensity measurements are carried out. For a two-colour system, we first unite the target region detected from the red channel and the target region detected from the green channel. The reason is simple both probes were hybridized to the same target, so if one observe *either* one of them, the underlying region must belong to original target. The probe intensity measurement is chosen to be the average gray level within the target region. Keeping in mind that the final measurement is the ratio of two intensities (R/G), the average measurement will provide, to some degree, a data smoothing effect. The local background value is then subtracted from the reported probe intensities form the red channel (R) and the green channel (G); the ratio (R/G) is then calculated measurements. There are, of course, other choices for ratio measurement, including (I) the average of ratios from every pixel location, and (II) the linear regression slope of R-G gray-values from every pixel location.

Ratio Analysis

One can used expression ratio calculations to determine whether gene expression differs significantly between the red and green channels. Such an approach is intuitive because two similar samples lead to a R/G ratio close to 1. Assume the ratio (denoted as *i*) extracted from a microarray image satisfied the following conditions: (1) normality, (2) independence, (3) being sufficiently positive and (4) having a constant-coefficient-of-variation. We can approximate the ratio distribution as follows:

$$f_1(t) = \frac{(l+t)\sqrt{l+t_2}}{c\,(l+t^2)^2\sqrt{2\pi}}\; e^{\frac{(t-1)^2}{2c^2\,(l+t^2)}}$$

The distribution parameter can be estimated using a maximum likelihood method, and ratio calibration call be carried out by an interactive method (assuming that the two channels are not normalized). In order to satisfy the null hypothesis, which requires no intensity change from red to green, we have chosen a set of "housekeeping" genes. These genes have been selected and experimentally verified as being stable in most experiments (R/G) = 1.0). While being referred to as a "housekeeping" gene set, their selection is based on biology as well as on their experimental calculation across thousands of observations under numerous experimental conditions. This selection of a "house-keeping" set has been modelled by labelling the same mRNA sample from the same cell line (UACC-903) by both Cy3 and Cy5. The ratio distribution estimated by the actual data from the housekeeping set closely predicts the spread of the ratio (by parameter c). Furthermore, the peak of the ratio distribution is correctly calibrated to 1, which is what one can expect since the two samples should be essentially identical. The significance of basing our measurement on the analytical ratio distribution is that we can associate a confidence interval to each ratio measurement so that a significant difference can be easily detected. More importantly, this approach allows us to associate a *p*-value to each ratio measurement. Finally, it is possible to derive quality measurements from the above equation (5, 6).

Multiple Image Analysis (Gene Clustering)

The value of microarray technology is not only that it enables a fast screening method for the expression of individual genes, but also is that it enables the investigator to study gene interactions in parallel. While the previous discussion has focused on single-image (slide) analysis reports of genes with significantly different expression level between two probes, multiple images (slides) can be analyzed to explore the temporal expression pattern for a given gene, or to study the similarity between expression patterns from different samples (*e.g.*, patterns of expression between stages of cancer progression).

7. Pal, S.K., Ghosh, A. and Kundu, M.K. (2000). *Soft Computing for Image Processing*. Physica-Verlag, A Springer-Verlag Company.

8. Pal, S.K. and Mitra, S. (1999). *Neuro-Fuzzy Pattern Recognition: Methods in Soft Computing*. John Wiley and Sons Inc.

CHAPTER 9

DEVELOPMENT OF COMBO-VACCINE A New Trend

Introduction

Combo vaccine, combination of various vaccines, is the future trend which will replace the general vaccine (flight against specific single infecting agents or toxins or antigens) and by this one company will, enable to take the lead over other. This chapter discusses the available general vaccines and combo vaccines their covering areas. It also discusses the possibility of combo vaccine.

The dormant vaccine market saw its first spark with the launching of *Rabipur,* a rabies vaccine in 1986-87 mainly in India. It is dominating till date. Vaccines are traditionally prepared for the market with the objective of fight against specific infecting agents or toxins or antigens produced by them.

Most of the virus vaccines today are live attenuated strains that bestow profound immunity and stimulate the entire repertoire of immune response in the both humoral antibody and cell mediated (3). Local immunoglobulin at the mucosal surfaces is produced which help to prevent superficial replication of the virus and hence spread of infection to other individuals.

A trend to development of combo-vaccine, combination of various vaccine, mainly Hepatitis-B+DPT; Diphtheria + Tetanus + Pertusis + H influenza are the most important type of combo vaccine (1).

The combo vaccine (2) is more useful to reducing the number of injection which must be much welcomed by infants and patients.

Some Vaccine and Combo-vaccine

Some various vaccine type, their manufacture company and possible combo-vaccine are given below:

Rabies Vaccine (for Dog Bite)

Some types of Rabies vaccines are available in present market. Hvecnsk Company marketed purified chick embryo cell rabies vaccine as brand name *Rabipur,* Cadilla marketed inactivated rabies vaccines prepared on vero cells as brand name *Verorab.* Human deploid cell rabies vaccines are also available in brand name Si. No such combo rabies vaccine are available today.

Measles/Mumps and Rubella Vaccine

These type of vaccine are also available today from Serum and Pasteur Lab in brand named *Tresivac* and *Trimovac* respectively.

H-Influenza based Vaccines

H-influenza + Diphteria or Tetanus are also marketed today as a brand name *Hbitter* from Wyelth and *Hibest* from Pasteur Lab. H-influenza vaccines (type b) for H-influenza are available nowadays from Pasteur Lab named *Vaxigrip.*

Chickenpox Vaccines

These type of vaccine are also available today from SKB and Pasteur Lab. in brand named *Vailrix* and *Okavax* respectively.

Hepatitis Vaccine

Hepatitis is a contagious disease affecting liver and it is very common in India. Six types of hepatitis viruses have been identified, of which hepatitis A is responsible for common "jaundice". Almost all Indians are exposed to this virus "A". Hepatitis B are responsible for chronic liver disease and Hepato Cellular Carcinoma. This being reason to allure the pharmaceutical companies in India to enter in it. Today market dynamics has changed for this vaccine only. This has led to new emerging market.

Mainly Hepatitis A and Hepatitis B vaccines are available. Only one type Hepatitis A vaccine available *i.e., Harox* from SKB and so many Hepatitis B vaccine from SKB, Panacea Biotech, Shanta

FIGURE 9.1: Possible Combo-vaccine in Future

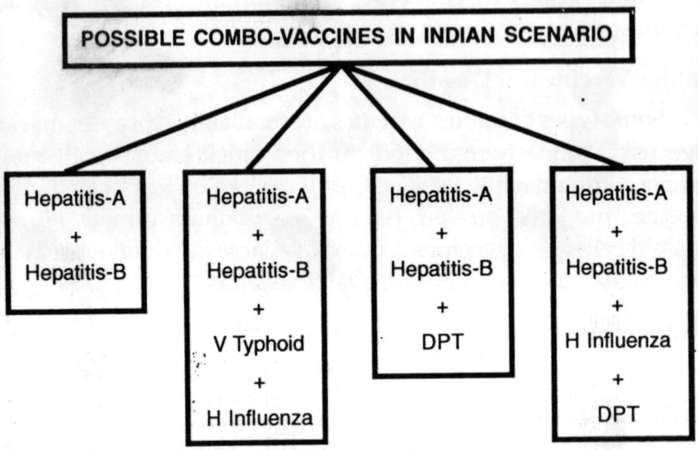

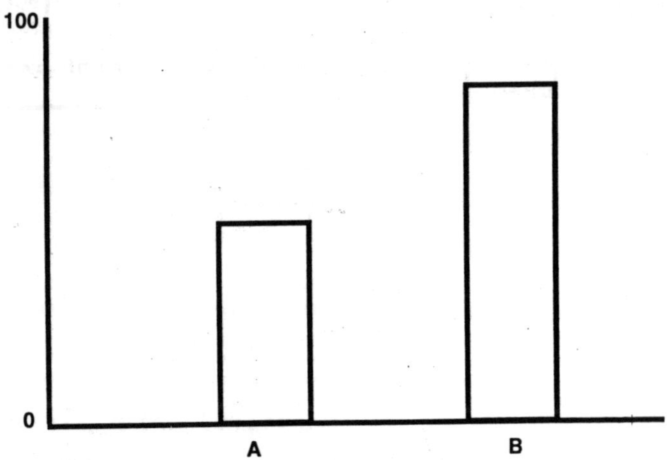

FIGURE 9.2: Comparison of needs (in the market) of (A) General Vaccine and (B) Combo Vaccine

Pharmaceutical, Intas, Wockhrdt, VH Vagat, Hepatitis vaccine have change the market dynamics.

Typhoid Vaccines

These type of vaccine are also available today from Hoechest, New Gen, and Pasteur Lab in brand named *Typhoral, Typhim* and *Typhivax* respectively.

New Classical Combo-Vaccine

Hepatitis B + DTP is anew combo-vaccine recently introduced by SKB, Diphtheria + Tetanus + Pertussis + H-Influenza (A type) is also available from W Lederle and Pasteur Lab as brand name *Tetramune* and *Tetra Hibest*. A new vaccine designed to protect children against six different illnesses appears to provide similar immunity as a combination of two separate vaccines is going to be marketed by Aventis Pasteur MSD as a brand name *Hexavac*. It is already approved for use in the European Union that provide immunity against diphtheria, tetanus, pertisus (whooping cough), polio, hepatitis B and haemophilus influenza B (Hib).

Conclusion

There are so many possibilities for new combo vaccine (Fig. 9.1). Laboratories are trying to development of new type of combo vaccine due to good demand in the market (Fig. 9.2). The combo-vaccine will change the entire pharma market scenario. The new type can be introduced for prophylaxis purpose. Company will enable to take the lead over other and overcome price barriers through these combo vaccine.

Despite the single dose vaccine, irritation at the injection site and mild side effects including irritability or unusual crying were significantly more common in combo- vaccine after the first dose, but not after second and third dose.

References

1. Srivastava, R.K. (2000). Hepatitis Vaccine: Setting New Standards in Marketing. *Exp. Phar. Pul.*, 7(1): 29.
2. Anonomous, S. (2001). Six-in-one Vaccine Safe and Effective. *Exp. Phar. Pul.*, 7(11): 22.
3. Reddi, O.S. (2000). DNA Vaccine. *Exp. Phar. Pul.*, 7(2): 23.

CHAPTER 10

CHROMATOGRAPHY The Most Effective Technique for Development of New Herbal Medicine

Introduction

Chromatographic techniques like gas liquid chromatography (GLC), high pressure liquid chromatography (HPLC) and high performance thin layer chromatography (HPTLC) have become the most important techniques for the characterization of herbal drugs. This chapter discusses the techniques for development of new herbal medicine and the importance HPTLC due to some advantage.

There has been a resurgence of interest in herbal medicine world wide in recent years. The need to device simple, yet effective protocols for standardization of the vast array of natural products, which are broadly classified as herbal medicines, has been bogging the mind of scientist. There can not be any singular approach to the standardization of herbal drugs because of many complexities involved. However, an attempt is being made to come out with a least level of standardization by analyzing the chemical components of what constitute 'herbal medicine'. Many difficulties are encountered in adopting a modern considerably in their components depend their part of herbal drugs. Natural products vary season, geographical locations and method of storage, drying etc. Individual herbal extracts have numerous constituents. Extraction process differ with respect to solvent used, time, temperature, pressure, technique etc. Manufacturing process vary from company to company. But the chromatographic techniques like gas liquid chromatography (GLC), high pressure liquid chromatography (HPLC) and high performance thin layer chromatography (HPTLC) have become the most important and frontline techniques for the characterization of herbal drugs.

The Techniques for Development of New Herbal Medicine

The standardization of herbal medicine involves using a herbs which is authenticated botanically and the bio-efficiency of it's extract is pharmacologically. Any pharmacological protocol developed for the purpose essentially has to combine the principles of modern pharmacology without compromising on the essentially holostic nature of herbal medicine. This extract becomes a reference standard. This reference drug extract can be either quantified for active principal or for the procedure involves standardizing a desirable extraction procedure. The second step involves resolving this extract by chromatography into as many fractions as possible. This highly resolved chromatogram is then scanned at 5 to 6 wavelength in UV, fluorescence and if possible in visible light, in order to get numerous peaks from the same chromatogram. This gives a chromatographic profile (fingerprint) for the extract. It is then necessary to record absorbance spectra of all the fractions. When comparing two of extracts, in fingerprinting approach, it is necessary that Rf and peak areas/height of reference and sample should be match. Secondly the spectra much also match.

HPTLC is a instrumental approach to TLC and involves automation in different stages of TLC. In HPTLC, protected aluminium sheets or glass plates are used, which are readily available commercially. Silica gel is the most commonly used absorbent in the HPTLC plates. HPTLC plates with modified layer like RP- 18, cynao, diol, amino, chiral etc are also available for specialized application.

Some common active ingredients present in herbal drugs, have been classified to belong to the primary groups like alkaloids, anthraglycosides, arbutin, bitterprinciples, cardiacglycosides, counmarins, phenols, carboxylic acids, essential oils, flavonoids, saponins and valepotriates. Rapid screening methods are now available to check for the presence of these components, either in crude extracts or in formulation.

Micro-preparative chromatography can be used either for preliminary cleanup procedures or for the isolation of marker compounds, which can subsequently be characaterize by mass spectroscopy or nuclear resonance.

Conclusion

Though there are so many technique like gas liquid chromatography (GLC), high pressure liquid chromatography (HPLC) and high performance thin layer chromatography (HPTLC) are important techniques for the characterization of herbal drugs. But in HPTCL, aluminium sheet or glass plates are readily available commercially. Simple clean up and extraction process are minimal in HPTLC as these plates being disposable there is no problem of contamination. This result is considerable saving of time and cost. It is a completely visual technique and post-chromatographic derivation is an important part of visualizing constituent. The developed HPTLC plates are visualized in UV cabinets for preliminary detection and then scanned by HPTLC scanners. Modern HPTLC scanners are equipped denterium tungsten and mercury lamps for the measurement of the compound in their ultraviolet, visible and fluorescence modes. So, HPTLC may be the best technique than others for the development of new herbal medicine.

References

1. Bharat, S. (2000). Role of HPTLC in Standardization of Herbal Medicine. *Exp. Phar. Pul.*, 7(6): 11-12.

2. Mazaraki, J. (2000). Pharmaceutical Analysis by HPLC. *Exp. Phar Pul.*, 7(6): 17.

3. Telange, R.P. (2000). Application of Gas Chromatographic Headspace Analysis. *Exp. Phar. Pul.*, 6(35): 11.

CHAPTER 11

TRANSGENIC TECHNOLOGY Modern Factories for Synthesis of New Molecule

Introduction

Transgenic technology will be one of the most important technology for pharmaceutical industry. Transgenic animals or plants will be used as 'factories' for synthesis of the new pharmaceutical molecules. This chapter discusses the procedure for production of transgenic animal or plants for molecular farming and their present and future for pharmaceutical technology.

A major goal of biotechnology industry is also the use of transgenic animals or plants as 'factories' for manufacturing of pharmaceuticals products. Large scale production of valuable proteins from transgenic animals or plants from their by products like milk, blood, urine etc. which will be used as a pharmaceutical products after extraction is also known as 'molecular farming' (1) or 'bio-reactors' (2).

Production of Transgenic Animal or Plants for Molecular Farming

The transgenic technology includes the isolation of a gene for specific protein, transfer of that particular gene into new plant or animal embryo, implementation of embryo in field (for plant) or uterus of female (for animal), allow them for development, expression of the gene and extraction of the protein in large amount for pharmaceutical use. Isolation of a gene for a specific protein that can be done through various steps which is sited in (Figure 2.1 in Chapter 2).

Gene transfer can be done through various methods like electroporation, gene gun, microinjection, biolistics mediated gene transfer, liposome mediated gene transfer, gene transfer using chemical methods and vector mediated genetransfer. In plants mainly vector is used gene transfer. But in animals, microinjection method is popular Electroporation, liposome are also use in some laboratory. Microinjection of DNA into plant nucli is more difficult than in animal cells.

Transgenic Technology Present and Future

Scientist has achieved considerable skills and efficiency in introducing exogenous or foreign genes whose stable expression in targeted animals or plants give rise transgenic individual. The concept of 'bio-reactors' through transgenic organisms was Thompson Institute for plant research, Ithaca, New York, when they tried introducing genes encoding antigen of bacterial and viral pathogens which can be get expressed in plants in a form where they remain native, immunogenic properties (3). The effect was stimulated by interest in evolving capacity of organism to produce different class of pharmaceutical value. Recently the most important indication of transgenic study is the possibility of using fish as 'bio-reactors' to produce pharmaceutical product human insulin which has been explored recently by Wright's team in Halifax (Table 11.2). The team injected human insulin gene into a fish (tilapia) for production of human insulin (4). Now some targeted proteins of pharmaceutical interest and their specific genes are already being isolated. Those recombinant therapeutic proteins will be the new molecules for pharmaceutical industry, which will be synthesis through transgenic technology (Table 11.1).

TABLE 11.1: Some Recombinant Therapeutic Proteins Future from the Transgenic Technology

Recombinant Proteins	*Applications*
Tumar Necrotic Factor (TNF)	Used as anticancer and antiviral agent.
Interleukin-2 (ILO2).	Used as anticancer and antiviral agent.
Interferons (IFN).	Used as anticancer and antiviral agent.
Human Protein C.	Anti-coagulant regulator of haemostasis.
Human Factor IX.	Clotting factor for haemophilia B.
Human Factor VII.	Clotting factor for haemophilia A.
Hepatitis B Surface Antigens.	Vaccine against hepatitis B.

TABLE 11.2: A List of Transgenic Mouse and Fish Produce and the Promoter, Enhancer and Structural Transgenes involve in each case

Animal	*Gene Transfer*
Fish	RGh, hGH, mMT/bGal, SV/hygro, AFP, bGal, dCry, mMT/hGH.
Mouse	mMT/rGH, mMT/ltGH, mMT/oGH, mMT/hGRF.

h-Human, m=Mouse, b=Brovine (ox), r=Rat, o=Ovine, c=Chicken

List of gene abbreviations

GH=Growth Hormone, MT=Metallothionein, Gal=Galactosidase, SV=SV40, hygro=Hygromicine, AFP=antifreeze protein, dCry=delta crystalline protein, GRF=Growth Releasing Factor

Promoter or enhancer is separated from stural gene by a slash (/).

References

1. Gupta, P.K. *Elements of Biotechnology*. Rastogi and Company, Meerut, India, 602 pp.
2. Chakraborty, Chiranjib and Haque, S. (2000). Edible Vaccine from Transgenic Fish. *Fishing Chimes*, 20(1): 104-105.
3. Masood, S., Rizvi, H. and Sing, R.P. (1996). Edible Vaccines from Transgenic Plants. *Physio. Mol. Biol Plants*, 5: 101-102.

4. Mackenzine, D. (1996). Doctors Farm Fish for Insulin. *New Scientist*, 20: 2056.

5. Mason, H.S., Lam, D.M.K. and Arntzen, C.J. (1992). *Boyce Thompson Institute for Plant Research*. Ithacn, New York.

CHAPTER 12

CLINICAL TRIALS
The Ultimate Testing Ground for Newly Prepared Drugs

Introduction

Clinical trials are the ultimate testing ground of a newly developed drug, to know whether the drug is fulfilling the proposed objective or not. There are four phase for clinical trials, those are phase I, II, III, IV. Clinical trials could be divided as Controlled trials and Uncontrolled trials. These are three main controlled trial designs – matched pairs, cross over design, mixed design. All are described briefly in this chapter.

Clinical trials are the test undertaken in both hospital and general practice centers in all therapeutic areas. Clinical trials are conducted in human beings to confirm the useful properties of new drugs which are predicted during pre-clinical studies. In simple words, the objective is to produce new knowledge from every patient's experience with the new medicine is essential from a clinical trial.

A clinical trial is a carefully and ethically designed experiment with the aim of answering some precisely framed questions. It has also been defined as scientific experiment in which a drug or procedure is applied with diagnositic, therapeutic or prophylactic intent to patient (1-4).

Methods of Clinical Trials

Clinical trials activity is generally considered under four phases. Healthy volunteers are used in phase II, III, IV used patients with varying degree of illness. It is extremely important to take the informed consent from both healthy individuals and patients before any trials.

Phase-I Studies

Following adequate animal studies, the first trial in human is considered in healthy volunteers. This study establishes that the new compound can be safely administered to human subjects. It establishes doses, duration of action, absorption, distribution, metabolism and excretion of the test drug.

Phase-II Studies

In these studies patients are used for the first time. The primary objective of these is to examine whether a new drug is effective for one (or more) clinical indications. Early studies during phase-II may be uncontrolled but they contribute valuable information. In this phase the pharmacokinetic effect of the drug are studied in patients as they may handle the drug differently due to modified body function.

During this phase early trials are started with single small dose with a few patients who are carefully monitored. Later multiple doses are employed and patient population are built. The doses used a series must be uses, establishes the therapeutic level and the maximum tolerated dose.

Phase-III Studies

These studies are started when the clinical researchers are convinced that an acceptable risk profile in relation to efficacy exist. During this period different types of trial designs are used. At the end of this phase, indications and dosage of drug are confirmed so that the drug can be given safely, even for prolonged used when indicated.

Phase-IV Studies

These studies include all the work which is undertaken after obtaining the manufacturing and marketing permission.

Clinical trials always involve making comparison. The most important considerations the design of a clinical trials. Basically clinical trials could be divided as controlled trials and uncontrolled trials.

Uncontrolled Trials (Open Trials)

Useful information can be obtained by well-planned and conducted uncontrolled studies, also known as open trials. Early phase-II studies may be conducted as uncontrolled open trials (*i.e.* both patients and doctors are aware they are using a new medicine). In these trials the effect of expectation or bias always remains. However one can say that open trials are unreliable and inaccurate. But open trials are relatively simple to setup and have important part to play in initiating studies of particular therapeutic diagnosis.

Controlled Trials

These trials compare the new drug against placebo or an established drug or treatment. There are three main controlled trial designs– matched pairs, cross over design, mixed design.

Matched Pairs

An attempt made to standardize the patient matching for series of physical social characteristic (*e.g.* age, sex and class). Alternately only patients with a particular

Cross Over Design

In this design patient is in his own control. A group of patient is Selected and given two or three regiments for a set period of time. This method can not be used where one of the drug curative or diseasc itself is self limiting.

Treatment period	*1*	*2*	*3*
Patient 1	A	B	C
Patient 2	B	C	A
Patient 3	C	A	B

This method enables a valid comparison between trials to be made.

Mixed Design

Here matched pair can be selected, treated with one medicine and then cross over. These trials could either be placebo controlled or against one or two established drugs. Placebo controlled trials are not meaningful when the diseases in itself limiting (*e.g.* toothache, peptic ulcer).

Conclusion

The question that are proposed to be answered are first framed. It makes the first step in the preparation of protocol. A protocol is a detailed statements of the plan of the clinical trials (Fig. 12.1). It is the most vital thing to eventual success of the trial.

A trial is usually consulted before starting the trial since it is very important to know as to how many patients should be taken up to get a positive answer to the questions that were framed. It is often

FIGURE 12.1: Protocol for Clinical Trials (*Used in Internal Documents)

Protocol

- Objective of the study
- Number of patients to be included
- Criteria for selection fo patients
- **Design of study**
- Duration of the study
- **End points to be used**
- Laboratory studies-haematological and biochemical
- Recording of result and adverse reactions
- Total drug/comparative drug/placebo needed*
- Expense involved*
- Target date*

found that the trials suffer from to few patients to many, especially when the investigator lacks in statistical knowledge, has publication mania and holds an eminent position. The report of a not properly conducted trial may get published in a journal. Another thing remembers is that a superbly conducted trial may fail if the patient did not take the drug. Monitoring the drug consumption is extremely important for the success of a trial.

References

1. Jagota, S.C. and Jagota, P. (2001). Clinical Trials: The Ultimate Testing Ground for Drugs. *Exp. Phar. Pul.*, 7(12): 8.
2. Meltha, R.M. (1997). Pharmaceuticals I. Vallabh Prakasham, New Delhi, 420 pp.
3. Ali, A. and Mahamuni, A.D. (1997). Pharmaceuticals II. Vallabh Prakasham, New Delhi, 304 pp.
4. Kulkarni, S.K. (1999). Experimental Pharmacology. Vallabh Prakasham, New Delhi, 404 pp.

CHAPTER 13

GENE THERAPY A Revolutionary Development in Medicine

Introduction

Gene therapy is defined as the introduction of DNA or RNA into the cells with an objective of clinical benefit either prophylactic or therapeutic. Introduction can take place *in vitro* or *in vivo*. The later is cell therapy. The genes transferred in gene therapy are called transgenes.

Gene therapy is a revolutionary development in medicine since it is a very unique intervention programme resulting in the production of biological effects more potent and localised in appropriate cells or tissue for clinical benefit. It is limited to conditions where there is no therapy at present. The most obvious candidate diseases are various cancers, monogenic inherited disorders. HIV infection, cardiovascular conditions, rheumatoid arthritis cubital tunnel syndrome (1-6).

Process of Gene Therapy and Vector

For the introduction of a gene into the appropriate target cell or tissue delivery systems are needed to carry the gene. There are three main types of vehicles – viral, non-viral and physical systems. At present, the viral systems are considered to be more efficient and most ongoing trials involve the use of viral vectors. These viruses are Adenovirus and Adeno-associated virus (AAV). The other delivery system involves the delivery of naked DNA condensed on cationic polymers or cationic lipid or anionic liposomes (6). Electroporation biolestic (particle bombardment) are also under study.

For human gene therapy, AAV vectors have to generate a high titre around 10^{10}. A wide variety of human cells and cell lines have been transduced *in vitro* by AAV vectors. Human blood cells like CD 34^{+} may be a difficult target. Most studies with AAV vectors have focussed on direct *in vitro* delivery. These vectors have produced to be highly useful in providing long term gene expression *in vivo*, targeting slowly proliferating of post mitotic and non-dividing cells. These are the best targets for AAV gene therapy.

AAV vectors expressing CFTR cDNA (cystic fibrosis trans-membrane receptor) were delivered by bronchosocopy to the airway epithelium in lungs of rabbits and human primates brain of AAV vectors expressing receptor gene or Tyrosine Hydroxylase (an enzyme) mediated gene expression for 3-6 months. Prolonged persistence of therapeutic levels were achieved in human Erythropoietin (EPO) by intra-muscular injection of AAV human EPO vector. *In vitro* studies prove that therapeutic levels of gene expression can be achieved. There has been so far no ill effects.

Disease for Somatic Gene Therapy

Blame genes too susceptibilities to rheumatiod arthritis, schizophrcllin, manic-depressive psychosis, juvenile disease and many more. The most promising therapeutic approach is in cancer therapy which has resisted treatment all these decades. There are also some other discases need to gene therapy which is recorded in Table 13.1.

Cellular Target for Somatic Gene Therapy

Now some cellular targets (4) have been explored for gene therapy are:

Bone Marrow-totipotent Stem Cell

Bone marrow are readily accessible for experimental manipulation, Totipotent stem cell give rise to red blood cells, T cells, B cells neutrophils, eostinophils, basophils, macrophages, kupfer cells, platelets.

TABLE 13.1: Some Diseases for Somatic Gene Therapy

Diseases	*Current Therapy*
Severe Combined Immunodeficiency	Bone Marrow Transplantation
Phenolketonuria	Restriction of Dietary Phenylalanine
Deficiency of Peptide Hormones	—
Thalassemia	Blood Transfusion
Sickle Cell Diseases	Blood Transfusion.
Cystic Fibrosis	Antibiotics, Physical Cleaning of Lungs
Emphysema	Replacement Therapy, Lowering Environmental Risks
Hemophilia A	Concentrate of Factor VII by Transfusion
Gaucher's Disease	Repair Bone Damage, Enzyme Replacement

Hepatic Cells

Hepatic cells is a difficult but important target for gene replacement therapy because many important metabolic and synthetic function are associated with liver.

Fibroblast

Fibroblast are interesting targets for gene therapy because it can be easily harvested, grown in culture and transformed with recombinant virus.

Endothelium and Pulmonary Epithelium Cells

Pulmonary epithelial and endothelium of many organs sucl as blood vessels, intestine, pancreatic ducts, bile ducts are importan for gene therapy because they are readily available for infection by retroviruses *in vivo* and are also capable of substantial proliferation.

Endocrine Cells

Endocrine cells will be targets for therapy because of various endocrine and metabolic deficiency states.

Central Nervous System

There are several diseases in which a brain is affected organ. Introduction of gene into neurons in central nervous system is currently being studied.

Smooth Muscle Cells of Blood Vessel Walls

Smooth muscles cells of blood vessel walls are considered for ex vivo gene therapy because they are in contact with the circulatory system.

Conclusion

Although the skill of gene therapy in the nascent infant stages of development, it offers the possibility for major advances in the prevention and treatment of diseases. We do complete that increased collaboration among physicians, molecular biologist and cells biologist will result in the development of highly integrated approach to this new form of therapy (Table 13.1). It may be a day where pills impregnated with generic material might be a practicable and cost effective strategy for even relatively mild disorders such as lactase deficiency (3).

None of these developments is yet conclusive albeit they are significant first step towards a goal that could ultimately give man, the power to play god. What will we do with that kind of power? It is for the scientific community to provide a suitable answer.

References

1. Reddi, O.S. (2000). Gene Therapy in Cardiomyopathy Treatment. *Exp. Phar. Pul.*, 6(29): 22.
2. Anonymas, A. (2000). Gene Therapy: Is the Future? *Exp. Phar. Pul.*, 6(33): 2.
3. Menji, S. and Soohinda, B.S. (2001). Clarion Call of a New Era. *Exp. Phar. Pul.*, 7(11): 8.
4. Jogdand, N.S. (1997). Human Gene Therapy. In: *Gene Biotechnology*, Himalaya Publishing House, Mumbai, pp. 298-307.
5. Anonymas, A. (2000). Gene Therapy Research Targets Muscular Dystrophy. *Esp. Phar. Pul.*, 7(3): 28.
6. Reddi, O.S. (2000). Advances in Biotechnology Gene Therapy. *Exp. Phar. Pul.*, 6(38): 2.

CHAPTER 14

Liposomes as Drug Delivery System for Biotechnological Drugs

Introduction

Liposomes were discovered in the mid 1960s (1) and originally studied as cell membrane models. They have since gained recognition in the field of drug delivery. Liposomes are formed by the self-assembly of phospholipid molecules in an aqueous environment. Shown schematically in Figure 14.1(a), the amphiphilic-phospholipid molecules form a closed bilayer sphere in an attempt to shield their hydrophobic groups from the aqueous environment while still maintaining contact with the aqueous phase via the hydrophilic head group. The resulting closed sphere may encapsulate aqueous soluble drugs within the central aqueous compartment or lipid soluble drugs within the bilayer membrane. Alternatively, lipid soluble drugs may be complexed with cyclodextrins and subsequently encapsulated within the liposome aqueous compartment (2). The encapsulation within/association of drugs with liposomes alters drug pharmacokinetics, and this may be exploited to achieve targeted therapies.

Liposomes as Vaccine Adjuvants

Liposomes have been firmly established as immunoadjuvants (enhancers of the immunological response), potentiating both cell mediated and humoral immunity (3). Liposomal immunoadjuvants

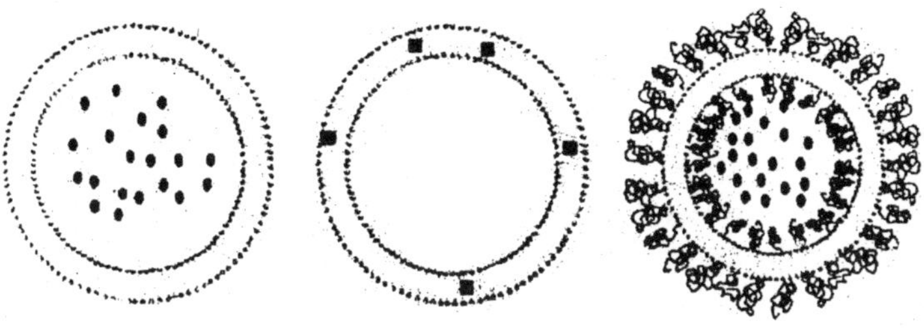

(A) (B) (C)

FIGURE 14.1: Liposomes. (A) Aqueous Soluble Drug Encapsulated in Aqueous Compartment; (B) A Hydrophobic Drug in the Liposome Bilayer; (C) Hydrophilic Polyoxyethylene Lipids Incorporated into Liposome

act by slowly releasing encapsulated antigen on intramuscular injection and also by passively accumulating within regional lymph nodes (4). Strategies that enhance the targeting of liposomes to regional lymph nodes, for example the use of phosphatidylserine liposomes (5) may thus improve adjuvanticity. Liposomal vaccines can be made by associating microbes, soluble antigens, cytokines or deoxyribonucleic acid (DNA) (6) with liposomes, the latter stimulating an immune response on expression of the antigenic protein (6). Liposomes encapsulating antigens which are subsequently encapsulated within alginate lysine microcapsules (7) to control antigen release, improve the antibody response. Liposomal vaccines may also be stored dried at refrigeration temperatures for up to 12 months and still retain their adjuvanticity (8).

Active Targeting of Liposomes

Immunoliposomes

The production of stealth liposomes, which are not rapidly cleared by the liver and spleen, made the active targeting of liposomes a real possibility. Various antibodies have thus been conjugated to the surface of stealth liposomes to produce immunoliposomes for active targeting, as opposed to the passively targeted species discussed above.

Stealth liposomes bearing an antibody that specifically binds intracellular myosin in ischaemic or necrotic cardiomyocytes targets infarcted areas in rabbits (9). The antibody dose not bind to cardiomyocytes with intact plasma membranes and hence avoids healthy tissue. The infarcted heart antibodies were attached to the liposome surface as shown in and the effectiveness of the antibody in homing the liposome found to be directly related to the level (10, 11) and molecular weight (12) of polyoxyethylene on the surface. A high polyoxyethylene density and polyoxyethylene with a molecular weight in excess of 2000 hampers the directing ability of the antibody by shielding the antibody from its target. To overcome this masking effect, surface antibodies such as the OX26 transferring antibody and a lung endothelial cell antibody (13) may be attached to the distal ends of polyoxyethylene chains. This attachment of antibodies improves the targeting ability when compared with the attachment of antibodies to the surface of non-stealth liposomes (13). This indicates that the extended circulation time achieved by stealth liposomes improves targeting simply because the prolonged circulation allows an extended period of time for liposomes to make contact with their target. Additionally, the exposure of antibodies to the target is enhanced by their attachment to the distal ends of the polyoxyethylene chains. Antibody Fab fragments attached to the distal ends of polyoxyethylene chains in stealth (14) or the liposome surface of non-stealth (15, 16) liposomes may also be used to target liposomes to solid tumours.

Although the stealth immunoliposomes with antibodies conjugated to the distal ends of polyoxyethylene chains are effective targeting agents, the conjugation accentuates the immune response to the antibody (17). This could ultimately result in the liposomes being cleared from the circulation prematurely, a feature that could limit the clinical development of these immunoliposomes. Unfortunately, although elegant science, anticancer drug targeting with immuno-stealth liposomes (18) and immunonon-stealth, liposomes (19) does not improve the tumoricidal activity when compared with ordinary stealth and non-stealth liposomes not bearing immunotargeting moieties. It is possible that a high binding of immunoliposomes to the periphery of solid tumours prevents their penetration into deeper layers (20). Alternatively, the lack of an incremental improvement in tumoricidal activity with immuno-targeted species could indicate that the extravasation of stealth liposomes is the rate limiting step to their accumulation at tumour sites (21). A further innovative utilisation of immunoliposomes involves a form of antibody directed enzyme prodrug therapy (ADEPT). The use of antibodies to direct prodrug activating enzymes to tumour tissue is the principle behind ADEPT (22) as discussed below. ADEPT type liposomes bearing antibodies and enzymes on their surface may be used to localise enzymes at the tumour site before administration of a prodrug. *In vitro*, prodrugs of epirubicin (23)and daunorubicin (22) may be activated by pre-treating cells with liposomes bearing cell specific antibodies and prodrug specific enzymes. The density of surface enzyme directly influences the tumoricidal activity of the drug and hence these rather complex systems must be carefully titrated to produce an effective formulation. While most immunoliposomes have been developed to target potentially toxic cancer chemotherapeutic agents, they may also prove beneficial in the treatment of other pathological conditions. The conjugation of interleukin 2 (IL-2) to the surface of non-stealth liposomes allows the targeting of toxic immunosuppressants to areas of the immune system participating in graft rejection, such as T-cells expressing the IL-2 receptor, (24) without affecting other parts of the immune system.

Limitations to the clinical use of immunoliposomes include a failure to demonstrate an advantage in experimental cancer chemotherapy plus the fact that these systems are rather complex. Each antibody disease state combination requires a specially tailored carrier (25) and specialised manufacture to retain the activity of the antibody.

Ligand Bearing Liposomes

An alternative targeting strategy that may ultimately have a wider application than the antibodies described above utilises surface moieties that are upregulated in certain diseases as targets. These include the folate receptor, over-expressed in ovarian carcinoma, and the cell adhesion molecules (*e.g.*, selectins and integrins), which are implicated in metastatic events. Liposomes bearing specific ligands such as folate may be used to target ovarian carcinomas, while specific peptides or carbohydrates may be used to target integrins and selectins (25). Targeting with small ligands appears more likely to succeed than the use of antibodies since these ligands are easier to handle and manufacture. Specifically, hamycin liposomes bearing mannosyl human serum albumin, which directs them to macrophages *in vivo*, are superior at suppressing leishmanial parasites than non-targeted liposomes (26). Hence, although liposomes are rapidly cleared by macrophages *in vivo*, an enhancement of this macrophage uptake by the use of targeting ligands results in an enhancement of the antileishmanial activity. Liposomes may also be targeted to hepatocytes by conjugating with asialofetuin (27). Such liposomes may be useful in the delivery of genes to hepatocytes for the treatment of specific diseases.

Liposomes in Gene Delivery

Human genome characterisation and recombinant DNA technology have created opportunities for gene therapy that previously never existed. Target diseases for such technology include certain cancers, (28) arteriosclerosis (29) cystic fibrosis (30) haemophilia, sickle cell anaemia and other genetic diseases. In addition, genes encoding for various antigens may be administered as vaccines.

The administration of the gene of interest should theoretically result in the expression of the therapeutic protein. However, the delivery of the large anionic bioactive DNA across cell membranes is by no means a simple feat. DNA is easily degraded by circulating and intracellular deoxyribonucleases and also must be delivered intact across the cell and nucleolar membranes to the nucleus. Liposomes have been used to achieve efficient intracellular delivery of DNA. Such liposomes are prepared from phospholipids with an amine hydrophilic head group (31). The amines may be either quaternary ammonium, tertiary, secondary or primary and the liposomes prepared in this way are commonly referred to as cationic liposomes, because they possess a positive surface charge at physiological pH. The use of cationic liposomes as gene delivery systems was pioneered in the late 1980s when *in vitro* studies demonstrated that the complexation of genes with liposomes promoted gene uptake by cells *in vitro* (32). Since this time, cationic liposomes of varying description have been used to promote the cellular uptake of DNA with resultant therapeutic protein expression by various organs *in vivo*.

On intravenous injection, cationic liposomes are rapidly cleared from the blood and most of the protein expression is found in the lung, the first capillary bed encountered after IV administration.

Lung expression could be the result of the formation of liposomal aggregates on interaction with blood proteins, which would then become trapped in the tiny lung capillaries. Alternatively, the cationic liposomes could become opsonised with lung specific opsonins on IV administration and hence be directed to the lung. It is not clear which of these, if either, is responsible for the high protein expression observed in the lung endothelium.

The knowledge gained in the development of anticancer liposomes, such as the prolongation of liposome circulation using polyoxyethylene lipids, may be applied in the development of gene delivery liposomes in order to produce efficient carriers (33). This strategy should aid liposome targeting in gene delivery. Thus far, targeting efforts with cationic liposomal gene formulations have been few and far between. A rare example is the targeting to mouse hepatocytes by the portal vein administration of cationic liposome DNA complexes coated with chylomicron remnants (34). Such liposomes are specifically, taken up by the apolipoprotein receptor. However, these chylomicron remnant coated liposomes were not targeted to the hepatocytes on tail vein administration. Although clinical trials with liposomal gene delivery in cystic fibrosis patients have concentrated on administration via non-parenteral routes, (35, 36) for the obvious reason that the disease manifests itself in the alveolar epithelium, it may be possible to treat this condition by the intravenous administration of the replacement gene-liposome complex. This is because such a strategy results in gene expression in distal regions of the alveolar epithelium.

Liposomal DNA is superior to free DNA in the treatment of experimental tumours. A cationic liposome formulation of the human interleukin 2 (IL-2) gene improves the tumoricidal activity of IL-2 in experimental xenografts. Cell kill in this case is mediated by expression of the IL-2 cytokine, which stimulates natural killer (NK) cell activity. Efficient arterial gene transfer will be beneficial in the treatment of arteriosclerosis and gene transfer into porcine arteries, via catheter, is enhanced by complexing the gene with liposomes, (37). Additionally, IV injection into tumour-bearing mice of the gene for diphtheria toxin A-chain complexed with cationic liposomes significantly reduces tumour volume compared with untreated controls (38).

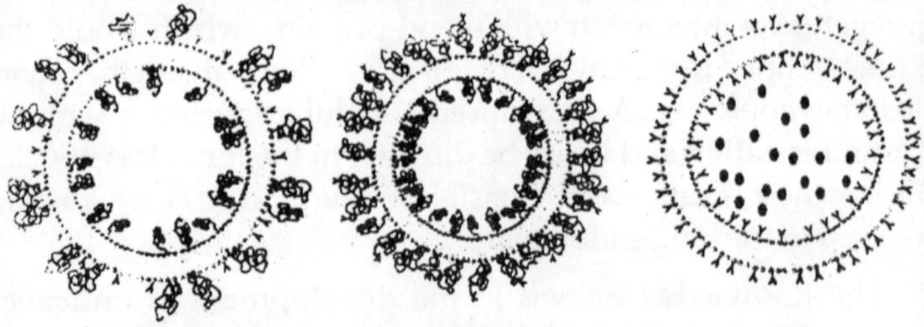

FIGURE 14.2: Immunoliposomes (A) Antibodies Attached to the Surface of Stealth Liposomes; (B) Antibodies Attached to the Distal Ends of Polyoxyethylene Chains in Stealth Liposomes; (C) Antibodies Attached to the Surface of Non-stealth Liposomes

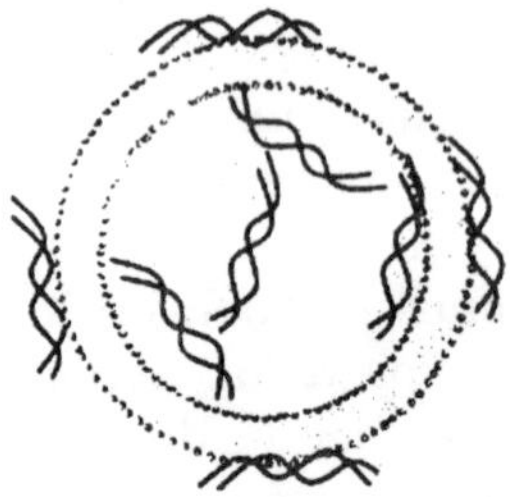

FIGURE 14.3: DNA-Liposome Complex

DNA vaccines administered as liposomal complexes also improve the antibody response over that seen with free DNA. Cell and humoral mediated immunity after the intramuscular administration of plasmids encoding for the S region of hepatitis B is enhanced by liposomal complexation. Cationic liposomes, by virtue of being able to transfer DNA more efficiently into cells than can be achieved with naked DNA alone, should lead to an increase in the level of antigen expression and hence an increase in the immune response to the antigen.

Although the experimental data indicate that cationic liposomes are able to facilitate the transfer of DNA into live mammalian cells, there are still major problems that need to be overcome in order to approach the ideal. These include a reduction in the rapid clearance

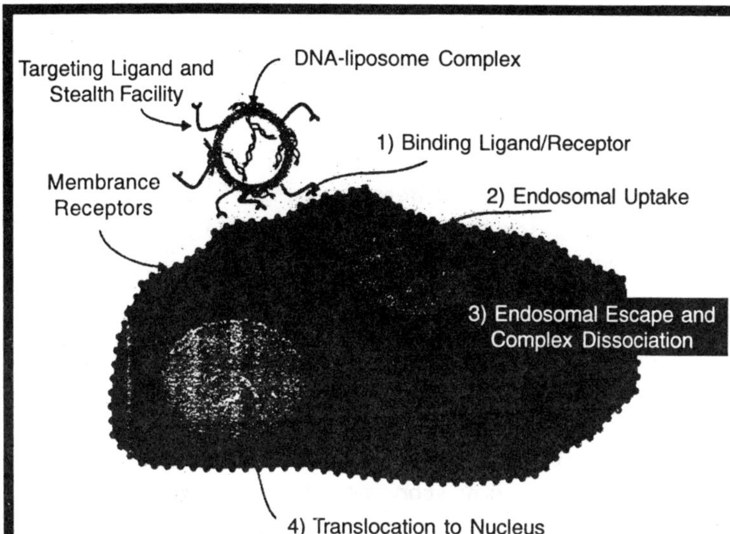

FIGURE 14.4: The Optimisation of Liposomal Gene Delivery

of cationic liposomes and the production of efficiently targeted liposomes. At the cellular level, the problems may be overcome by improving receptor mediated uptake using appropriate ligands, the endowment of liposomes with endosomal escape mechanisms, a more efficient translocation of DNA to the nucleus and the efficient dissociation of the liposome complex just before the entry of free DNA into the nucleus.

Non-ionic Surfactant Vesicles (Niosomes) and Other Synthetic Surfactant Vesicles

Niosomes

The success achieved with liposomal systems stimulated the search for other vesicle forming amphiphiles. Non-ionic surfactants were among the first alternative materials studied (39) and a large number of surfactants have since been found to self assemble into closed bilayer vesicles (40) which may be used for drug delivery.

Niosomes as Vaccine Adjuvants

Niosomal antigens are potent stimulators of the cellular and humoral immune response (41, 42). The formulation of antigens as a niosome in water-in-oil emulsion further increases the activity of antigens (43). The controlled release property of the emulsion formulation is responsible for enhancing the immunological response.

Liposomal drug delivery system is very effective for biotechnological drugs. Alteration of the liposome surface is necessary in order to optimize liposomal drug targeting for different biotechnological drugs.

References

1. Bangham, A.D., Standish, M.M., Watkins, I.C. (1996). Diffusion of univalent ions across lamellae of swollen phospholipids. *J. Mol. Biol.*, 13: 238-252.

2. McCormack. B., Gregoriadis, G. (1994). Drugs-in-cyclodextrins-in-liposomes: A novel concept in drug-delivery. *Int. J. Pharm.*, 112: 249-258.

3. Gregoriadis, G., Gursel, I., Gursel, M., McCormack, B. (1996). Liposomes as immunological adjuvants and vaccine carriers. *J. Control Rel.*, 41: 49-56.

4. Gregoriadis, G. (1995). Engineering liposomes for drug delivery: Progress and problems. *TI/Biotechnology*, 13: 527-537.

5. Oussoren, C., Storm, G. (1998). Targeting to lymph nodes by subcutaneous administration of liposomes. *Int. J. Pharm.*, 162: 39-44.

6. Gregoriadis, G., Saffie, R., Da Souza, I.B. (1997). Liposome mediated DNA vaccination. *FEBS Lett.*, 402: 107-110.

7. Cohen, S., Bernstein, H., Hewes, C., Chow, M., Langer, R. (1991). The pharmacokinetics of, and humoral responses to antigen delivered by microencapsulated liposomes. *Proc. Natl. Acad. Sci.*, USA, 88: 10440-10444.

8. Kim, C.K., Jeong, E.J. (1995). Development of dried liposome as effective immuno-adjuvant for hepatitis B surface antigen. *Int J. Pharm.*, 115: 193-199.

9. Torchilin, V.P., Trubetskoy, V.S., Milshteyn, A.M., Canillo, J., Wolf, G.L., Papisov, M.I. *et al.* (1994). Targeted delivery of diagnostic agents by surface modified liposomes. *J. Control Rel.*, 28: 45-58.

10. Klibanov, A.L., Maruyama, K., Beckerleg, A.M., Torchilin, V.P., Huang, L. (1991). Activity of amphipathic poly (ethylene glycol)-5000 to prolong the circulation time of liposomes depends on the liposome size and is unfavorable for immunoliposome binding to target. *Biochem. Biophys. Acta.*, 1062: 142-148.

11. Mori, A., Klibanov, A.L., Torchilin, V.P., Huang, L. (1991). Influence of the steric barrier activity of amphipathic poly (ethyleneglycol) and ganglioside GMI on the circulation time of liposomes and on the target binding of immunoliposomes *in vivo*. *FEBS Lett.*, 284: 263-286.

12. Maruyama, K., Takizawa, T., Yuda, T., Kennel, S.J., Huang, L., Iwatsuru, M. (1995). Targetability of novel immunoliposomes modified with amphipathic poly (ethylene glycols), conjugated at their distal terminals to monoclonal-antibodies. *Biochem. Biophys. Acta.*, 1234: 74-80.

13. Maruyama, K., Takizawa, T., Takahashi, N., Tagawa, T., Nagaike, K., Iwatsuru, M. (1997). Targeting efficiency of PEG-imrnunoliposome-conjugated antibodies at PEG terminals. *Adv. Drug Delivery Rev.*, 24: 235-242.

14. Maruyama, K., Takahashi, N., Tagawa, T., Nagaike, K., Iwatsuru, M. (1997). Immunoliposomes bearing polyethyleneglycol-coupled Fab' fragment show prolonged circulation time and high extravasation into targeted solid tumors *in vivo*. *FEBS Lett.*, 413: 177-180.

15. Crosasso, P., Brusa, P., Dosio, F., Arpicco, S., Pacchioni, D., Schuber, F. *et al.* (1997). Antitumoral activity of liposomes and immunoliposomes containing 5-fluorouridine prodrugs. *J. Pharm. Sci.*, 86: 832-839.

16. Nassander, U.K., Steerenberg, P.A., Dejong, W.H., Vanoverveld, W., Boekhorst, C., Poels, L.G. *et al.* (1995). Design of immunoliposomes directed against human ovarian-carcinoma. *Biochem. Biophys. Acta.*, 1235: 126-139.

17. Harding, J.A., Engbers, C.M., Newman, M.S., Goldstein, N.I., Zalipsky, S. (1997). Immunogenicity and pharmacokinetic attributes of poly (ethylene glycol) grafted immunoliposomes. *Ibid.* 1327: 181-192.

18. Goren, D., Horowitz, A.T., Zalipsky, S., Woodle, M.C., Yarden, Y., Gabizon, A. (1996). Targeting of stealth liposomes to erbB-2

(Her/2) receptor: *In vitro* and *in vivo* studies. *Br. J. Cancer*, 74: 1749-1756.

19. Vingerhoeds, M.H., Steerenberg, P.A., Hendriks, J., Dekker, L.C., vanHoesel, Q., Crommelin, D.J.A. *et al.* (1996). Immunoliposome-mediated targeting of doxorubicin to human ovarian carcinoma *in vitro* and *in vivo*. *Ibid*, 74: 1023-1029.
20. Forssen, E., Willis, M. (1998). Ligand-targeted liposomes. *Adv. Drug Del. Rev.*, 29: 249-271.
21. K.D., Sharma, S.K., Springer, C.J., Antoniw, P., Boden, J.A., Rogers, G.T., *et al.* (1991). Antibody prodrug therapy (ADEPT): Clinical report. *Dis. Markers*, 9: 233-238.
22. Vingerhoeds, M.H., Haisma, H.J., Belliot, S.O., Smit, R.H.P., Crommelin, D.J.A., Storm, G. (1996). Immunoliposomes as enzyme-carriers (immuno-enzymosomes) for antibody- directed enzyme prodrug therapy (ADEPT): Optimization of prodrug activating capacity. *Pharm. Res.*, 13: 604-610.
23. Vingerhoeds, M.H., Haisma, H.J., Vanmuijen, M., Vanderijt, R.B.J. Crommelin, D.J.A., Storm, G. (1993). A new application for liposomes in cancer-therapy immunoliposomes bearing enzymes (immuno-enzymosomes) for site-specific activation of prodrugs. *FEBS Lett.*, 336: 485-490.
24. Konigsberg, P.J., Godtel, R., Kissel, T., Richer, L.L. (1998). The development of IL-2 conjugated, liposomes for therapeutic purposes. *Biochem. Biophys. Acta.*, 1370: 243-251.
25. Zalipsky, S., Hansen, C.B., deMenezes, D.E.L., Allen, T.M.. Long-circulatlng, polyethylene glycol-grafted immunoliposomes. *J. Control Rel.*, 39: 153-161.
26. Egilmez, N.K., Cuenca, R., Yokota, S.J., Sorgi, F., Bankert, R.B. (1996). *In vivo* cytokine gene therapy of human tumour xenografts in SCID mice by liposome mediated delivery. *Gene Therapy*, 3: 607-614.
27. Feldman, L.J., Steg, G. (1997). Optimal techniques for arterial gene transfer. *Cardiovasc. Res.*, 35: 391-404.
28. Griesenbach, U., Chonn, A., Cassady, R., Hannam, V., Ackerly, C., Post, M., *et al.* (1998). Comparison between intratracheal and intravenous administration of liposome-DNA complexes for cystic fibrosis. *Gene Therapy*, 1998: 181-188.

29. Zabner, J. (1997). Cationic lipids used in gene transfer. *Adv. Drug Del. Rev.*, 27: 17-28.
30. Smith, J., Zhang, Y.L., Niven, R. (1997). Toward development of a non-viral gene therapeutic. *Ibid*, 26: 135-150.
31. Lasic, D., Templeton, N.S. (1996). Liposomes in gene therapy. *Ibid*, 20: 221-226.
32. Felgner, P.L., Gadek, T.R., Holm, M., Roman, R., Chan, H.W., Wenz, M. *et al.* (1987). Lipofection: A highly efficient, lipid-mediated DNA-transfection procedure. *Proc. Natl. Acad. Sci.*, USA, 84: 7413-7417.
33. Chonn, A., Cullis, P.R. (1998). Recent advances in liposome technologies and their applications for systemic gene delivery. *Adv. Drug Del. Rev.*, 30: 73-83.
34. Hara, T., Tan, Y., Huang, L. *In vivo* gene delivery to the liver using reconstituted chylomicron remnants as a novel nonviral delivery vector. *Proc. Natl. Acad. Sci.*, USA, 94: 1454-1452.
35. Porteous, D.J., Dorin, J.R., McLachlan, G., Davidson, Smith H., Davidson, H., Stevenson, B.J., *et al.* (1997). Evidence for safety and efficacy of DOTAP cationic liposome mediated CFTR gene transfer to the nasal epithelium of patients with cystic fibrosis. *Gene Therapy*, 4: 210-218.
36. Gill, D.R., Southern, K.W., Mofford, K.A., Seddon, T., Huang, L., Sorgi, F., *et al.* (1997). A placebo-controlled study of liposome-mediated gene transfer to the nasal epithelium of patients with cystic fibrosis. *Ibid*, 4: 199-209.
37. Stephan, D.J., Yang, Z.Y., San, H., Simari, R.D., Wheeler, C.J., Felgner, P.L., *et al.* (1996). A new cationic liposome DNA complex enhances the efficiency of arterial gene transfer *in vivo*. *Hum. Gene. Therapy*, 7: 1803-1812.
38. Watarai, T.S., Lee, J.T., Onuma, M., Ochiai, K., Kakidani, H., Yasuda, T. (1997). *In vivo* antitumour effect of cationic liposomes containing diphtheria toxin A-chain gene on cells infected with bovine leukemia virus. *J. Vet. Med. Sci.*, 59: 617-619.
39. Iga, K., Ohkouchi, K., Ogawa, Y., Toguchi, H. (1994). Membrane modification by negatively charged stearylpolyoxyethylene derivatives for thermosensitive liposomes: Reduced liposomal

aggregation and avoidance of reticuloendothelial system uptake. *J. Drug Target*, 2: 259-267.

40. Ahl, P.L., Bhatia, S.K., Meers, P., Roberts, P., Stevens, R., Dause, R., *et al.* (1997). Enhancement of the *in vivo* circulation lifetime of L-alpha-distearoylphosphatidylcholine liposomes: importance of liposomal aggregation versus complement opsonization. Biochem. Biophys. Acta., 1329: 370-382.
41. Brewer, J.M., Alexander, J. (1992). The adjuvant activity of nonionic surfactant vesicles (niosomes) on the Balb/C humoral response to bovine serum albumin. *Immunology*, 75: 570-575.
42. Hassan, Y., Brewer, J.M., Alexander, J., Jennings, R. (1996). Immune responses in mice induced by HSV-1 glycoproteins presented with ISCOMs or NISV delivery systems. *Vaccine*, 14: 1581-1589.
43. Yoshioka, T., Skalko, N., Gursel, M., Gregoriadis, G., Florence, A.T. (1995). A nonionic surfactant vesicle-in-water-in-oil (V/W/O) system: Potential uses in drug and vaccine delivery. *J. Drug Target*, 2: 533-539.

CHAPTER 15

STEM CELL A New Therapeutic Approach

A stem cell is a cell that has the ability to divide (self replicate) for indefinite periods- often throughout the life of the organism. Under the right conditions, or given the right signals, stem cells can give rise (differentiate) to the many different cell types that make up the organism. That is, stem cells have the potential to develop into mature cells that have characteristic shapes and specialized functions, such as heart cells, skin cells, or nerve cells.

The body uses different types of stem cells during development, maturation and adult life. *Embryonic stem cells* are only present during early development. These cells are responsible for the formation and maturation of all tissues and organs that make up the body. *Adult stem cells* are present in mature tissues throughout life. These cells are used to regenerate existing tissues, such as blood, skin and bone.

Different Stem Cells

Embryonic stem cells are derived from embryos shortly after fertilization. Fertilization occurs when a sperm and egg join to create a zygote. When the zygote begins to divide, it becomes a multi-celled embryo. Currently, most embryonic stem cell research is performed using embryos from laboratory mice. To study these cells, scientists create "cell lines", which are populations of dividing stem cells that

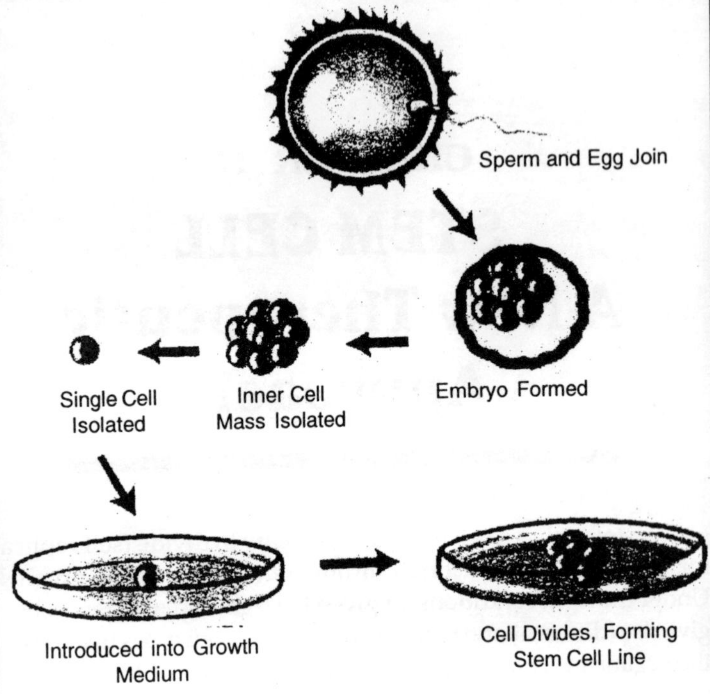

FIGURE 15.1: Creation of Stem Cell Line from an Embryo

originate from a single cell. To create an embryonic stem cell line, an embryo must be separated into individual cells. A single cell from the embryo is placed in a dish and provided with nutrients and growth factors that stimulate it to divide. The resulting cell line will continue to divide as long as it is kept in a highly controlled environment and provided with appropriate growth factors to prevent differentiation. To study how differentiation takes place, researchers treat the stem cells with different signalling factors and monitor the cells' responses.

Embryonic stem cells can also be derived from embryos created by *in vitro* fertilization (IVF). Usually, fertilization occurs within a woman's body, but IVF technology has made it possible to carry out fertilization and grow embryos in the laboratory. This technology

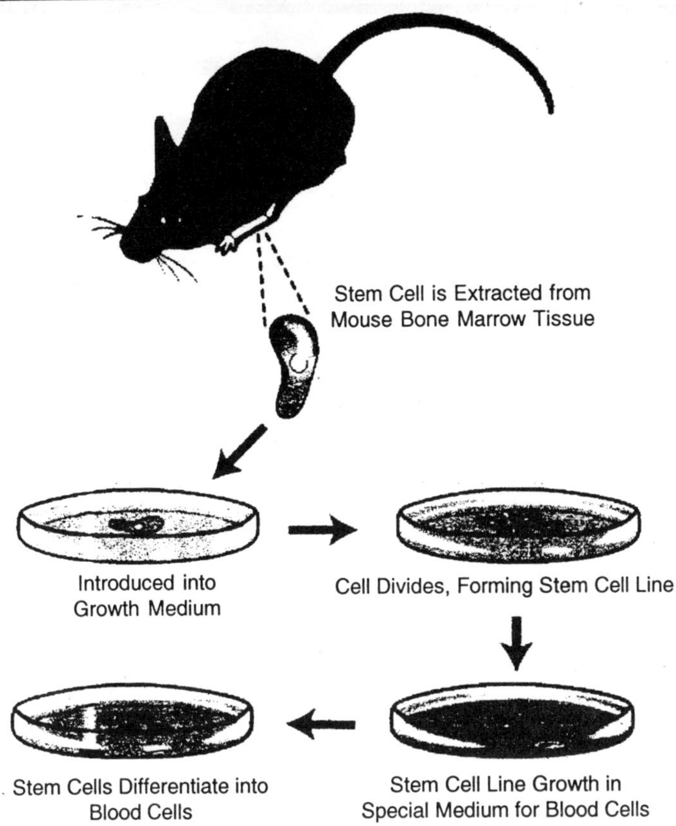

FIGURE 15.2: Creation of Stem Cell Line from Adult Tissue

has made it possible for many otherwise infertile couples to have children. In many cases, however, not all of the embryos created will be used, and the remaining embryos are frozen and stored. These embryos are potential resources for scientific research.

For therapeutic cloning, embryonic stem cells can also be created by the same procedure used to clone whole organisms, such as Dolly the sheep. Because of its potential medical uses, this method for creating stem cell is called "therapeutic cloning."

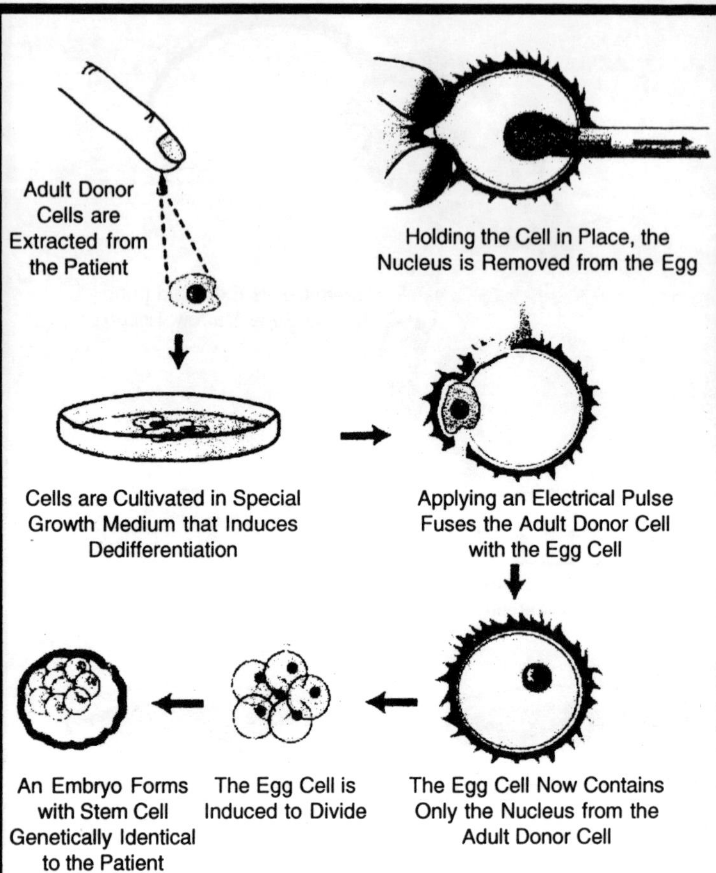

FIGURE 15.3: Therapeutic Cloning

In this procedure, a nucleus from an adult donor cell is inserted into a recipient egg cell from which the nucleus has been removed. The nucleus provides all of the necessary genetic information, in the form of DNA, for a cell to function and divide. The resulting cell is then stimulated to divide as a zygote would, resulting in the growth of embryonic stem cells that are genetically identical to the adult donor cell.

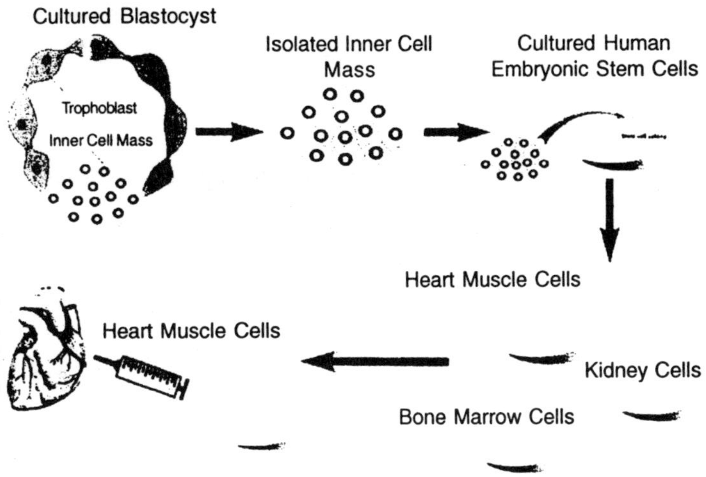

FIGURE 15.4: Culturing Human Embryonic Stem Cells

Therapeutic cloning might be a viable approach to growing an exact tissue match for a patient in need–if the donor nucleus came from the patient, the resulting embryonic stem cell line would be a perfect match.

Adult stem cells, isolated from mature tissues and cultured in the laboratory, are another excellent resource for research studies. Most research is performed using adult stem cells from model organisms such as rats and mice, since obtaining adult stem cells from humans would often involve invasive surgical procedures. Adult stem cells can differentiate into a large number of different cell types. For example, adult neural stem cells can differentiate into all of the types of cells normally found in the brain. Adult bone marrow stem cells can differentiate into blood, bone, muscle, cartilage, heart, liver and brain tissues. Scientists want to study both embryonic and adult stem cells to determine the potential for using both types in medical applications. Many scientists believe that embryonic stem cells are more versatile than adult stem cells.

Umbilical cord blood stem cells are obtained from the umbilical cords of newborn infants. These cells can be used in lieu of bone

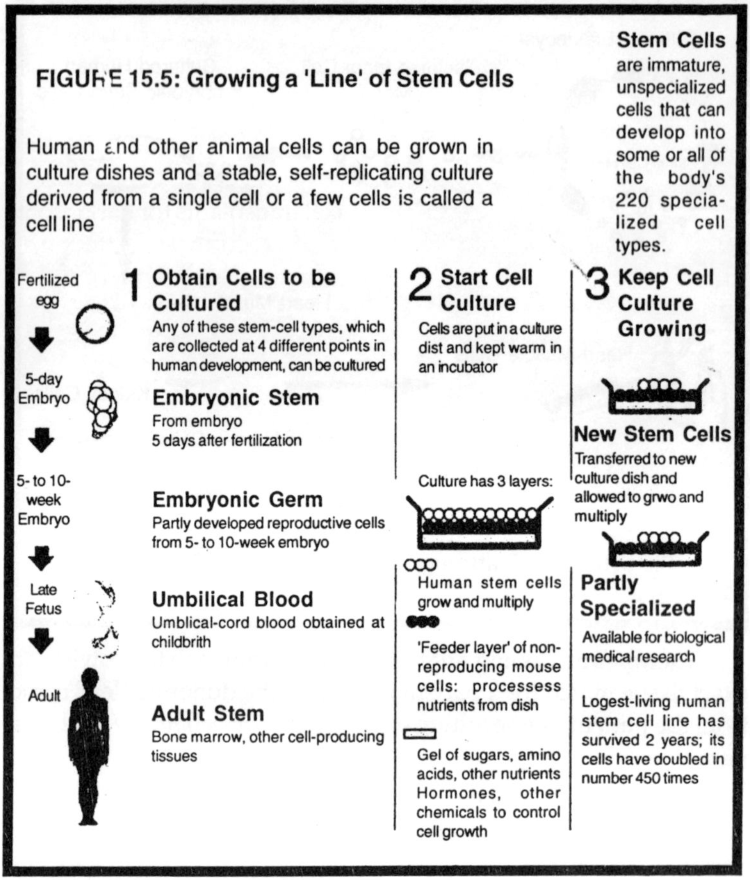

FIGURE 15.5: Growing a 'Line' of Stem Cells

marrow transplants to treat blood diseases such as leukemia, sickle cell anemia and Hodgkin's disease. Stem cells from umbilical cord blood can provide matching tissue for a family member needing a transplant.

Fetal stem cells are derived from aborted fetuses. Through experimental studies, fetal stem celis have been transplanted into the brains of patients with advanced Parkinson's disease, a disorder of the nervous system. The goal of the transplant is to replace nerve cells that have ceased to function properly, thus improving brain function; however, these studies have shown mixed results. Fetal stem cells may also be useful in treating other nervous system disorders and injuries.

Application of the Stem Cells

Researchers study stem cells to understand how development and differentiation pathways work. This allows them to investigate possibilities for repairing tissue damage caused by disease or injury, including:

1. Diseases that impair brain function, including Alzheimer's disease and Parkinson's disease
2. Spinal cord injuries
3. Blood diseases (including leukemia)
4. Diabetes
5. Heart disease
6. Limb amputation
7. Burns
8. Auto-immune diseases
9. Nerve diseases

Stem cells offer the opportunity of transplanting a live source for self-regeneration. Bone marrow transplants (BMT) are a well-known clinical application of stem cell transplantation. BMT can repopulate the marrow and restore all the different cell types of the blood after high doses of chemotherapy and/or radiotherapy, our main defense used to eliminate endogenous cancer cells. The isolation of additional stem and progenitors cells is now being developed for many other clinical applications. Several are described below:

Skin Replacement

The knowledge of stem cells has made it possible for scientists to grow skin from a patient's plucked hair. Skin (keratinocyte) stem cells reside in the hair follicle and can be removed when a hair is plucked (1). These cells can be cultured to form an epidermal equivalent of the patients own skin and provides tissue for an autologous graft, bypassing the problem of rejection. It is presently being studied in clinical trials as an alternative to surgical grafts used for venous ulcers and burn victims.

Brain Cell Transplantation

Neural stem cells were only until recently thought to be strictly embryonic. Many findings have proved this incorrect. The identification and localization of neural stem cells, both embryonic and adult, has been a major focus of current research. Potential targets of neural stem cell transplants include stroke, spinal cord injury, and neurodegenerative diseases such as Parkinson's disease. Parkinson's disease involves the loss of cells, which produce the neurotransmitter dopamine. The first double-blind study of fetal cell transplants for Parkinson's disease reported survival and release of dopamine from the transplanted cells and a functional improvement of clinical symptoms (2). However, some patients developed side effects, which suggested that there was an oversensitization to or too much dopamine. Although the unwanted side effects were not anticipated, the success of the experiment at the cellular level is significant. Again, further studies are needed and ongoing. Over 250 patients have already been transplanted with human fetal tissue.

Several biotechnology companies are developing different strategies of stem cell therapies.

1. *Diacrin* has been developing xenotransplants using fetal pig cells. Clinical trials for chronic stroke patients have begun. Presently, stroke patients require treatment within 24 hours after stroke for effective therapeutic results. Many patients do not receive treatment in time because the symptoms are not initially obvious. Diacrin's therapy could be applied weeks to months after the initial trauma.
2. *NeuroNova's* strategy is to culture adult human cells from donors, differentiate them in culture to produce the cell type (dopaminergic neurons), which is lost in Parkinson disease, and to transplant them into the brain of patients.
3. *Neurotech* is using genetically altered brain endothelial cells (engineered to produce human Interleukin-2) as immunotherapy for gliomas. Results from experiments in rats showed that these cells "mopped up" the tumour cells and as a result a clinical study has commenced.

Treatment for Diabetes

Diabetes affects 16 million people in the U.S. and is caused by the abnormal metabolism of insulin. Normally, insulin is produced and secreted by the cellular structures called the islets of Langerhans in the pancreas. Recently, insulin-expressing cells from mouse stem, cells have been generated (3). In addition, the cells self assemble to form structures, which closely resemble normal pancreatic islets and produce insulin. Future research will need to investigate how to optimize conditions for insulin production with the aim of providing a stem cell-based therapy to treat diabetes to replace the constant need for insulin injections.

Sources of Stem Cells

The main clinical application of stem cells is as a source of donor cells to be used to replace cells in transplantation therapy. Stem cells can be obtained from several sources:

Spare Embryos

Stem cells can come from leftover embryos stored at fertility clinics that were not used by couples to have children.

Special Purpose Embryos

Embryos are created *in vitro* fertilization (artificially in the lab) for the sole purpose of extracting their stem cells.

Cloned Embryos

Embryos are cloned in labs using somatic nuclear transfer method in order to harvest their stem cells.

Aborted Fetuses

Stem cells are taken from fetuses in early development that have been aborted.

Umbilical Cords

This after-childbirth tissue holds potential for research.

Adult Tissue or Organs

Stem cells are obtained from the tissue or organs of living adults during surgery.

Cadavers

Isolation and survival of neural progenitor cells from human post-mortem tissues (up to 20 hours after death) has been reported and provides an additional source of human stem cells (4).

Embryonic stem cells must be obtained when an embryo is in early development, that is, when the fertilized egg has divided to form about 1000 cells. These cells are separated and maintained in a cell culture dish, thereby halting embryonic development towards creating an individual. This is why embryonic stem cell research is the subject of ethical debates. Utilization of adult stem cells pose less of an ethical dilemma: however, adult stem cells may not have the same potential as those derived from embryos for medical therapeutics.

Our Expectations with Stem Cells

Today

Stem cells from bone marrow and umbilical cord blood are routinely and successfully used in treating leukemia and other blood diseases. Skin tissue is commonly grown in laboratories to supply skin grafts for burn victims. Finally, experimental studies have been performed to implant fetal cells in the brains of patients with advanced Parkinson's disease. While these studies show promise, it is not yet clear whether the therapeutic benefits of this treatment outweigh the risk of damaging side effects from the surgical procedure used to implant the cells.

Most medical breakthroughs using stem cells are still years away, however. The most, immediate goal is to figure out the true potential and limitations of both embryonic and adult stem cells, through basic research. Several promising findings have emerged from the study of model organisms such as mice and rats. For example, neural stem cells can restore body movement when implanted into the brains of rats with Parkinson's disease. Research has also shown that cells originating in one organ can travel to another and, assume the function of their new location. This phenomenon, called "plasticity," has been demonstrated in a number of cell types, including bone marrow cells, which can become liver or kidney, and brain cells, which can become blood or muscle.

In the Future

It may become possible for an individual to use a sample of his or her own stem cells to regenerate tissue, reducing or even eliminating the danger of tissue rejection. Alternatively, techniques such as therapeutic cloning might be used to create stem cells that are genetically compatible with the potential tissue recipient.

The current and future stem cell therapies described here rely on transplantation of cells into the body, where they would replenish or restore some lost function. But the greatest hope for stem cell research is that we will find ways to manipulate existing stem cells within the body to perform therapeutic tasks. In one such scenario, scientists might design a drug that directs a specific population of stem cells to restore a lost function. This approach would eliminate the need for invasive and risky surgical procedures to harvest and transplant stem cells.

Conclusion

The generation of new neurons in the adult brain is limited. However, self repair of neuronal cell death has been recently demonstrated in the mouse and suggests that stem cells which normally reside in the brain may someday be able to be stimulated by inducers in a manner similar to how we induce our immune system by vaccination (5). This would bypass the need for cell transplantation. Intensive research needs to be pursued into the cell mechanisms involved.

Scientists face technical, ethical and legal challenges in stem cell research. Scientists still have much to learn about stem cells and differentiation pathways. Some possible problems include the need to separate differentiated cells from stem cells, because injection of embryonic stem cells into the body can produce tumors. Also, in differentiated cells, misregulation of genes can lead to uncontrolled growth and tumor formation. Scientists don't yet have a good idea about how long a stem cell treatment might last, especially if adult stem cells are used instead of embryonic cells. Research is still inconclusive on whether manipulating the plasticity of cells will be a viable treatment option.

The news media have devoted much attention to ethical issues in stem cell research. These issues are important for society to consider. Should frozen embryos be granted the full moral status of a human being? What are the benefits of stem cell research? What are the risks?

Once society makes decisions about stem cells, by way of legislation or executive order, scientists have additional legal issues to address. We have already begun to make some of these decisions. In July 2001, the U.S. House of Representatives passed a bill that would ban human cloning. This measure also bans therapeutic cloning to create stem cells for research and medicine. Then, in August, President Bush issued a statement that supports research on existing embryonic stem cell lines, but stopped short of supporting the creation of new stem cell lines from existing embryos.

References

1. Jahoda, C. and Reynolds, A. (2000). Skin stem cells: A hairy issue. *Nature Medicine*, 6: 1095-1097.

2. Freed, C.R., Greene, P.E., Breeze, R.E., Tsai, W-Y., DuMoucel, W., Kao, R., Dillon, S., Winfield, H., Culver, S., Trojanowski, J.Q., Eidelberg, D. and Fahn, S. (2000). Transplantation of embryonic dopamine neurons for severe Parkinson's disease. *New England J. of Med.*, 344: 710-719.

3. Lumelsky, N., Blondel, O., Laeng, P., Velasco, I., Ravin, R., McKay, R. (2001). Differentiation of embryonic stem cells to insulin-secreting structures similar to pancreatic islets. *Science*, 292: 1389-1394.

4. Palmer, T., Schwartz, P.H., Taupin, P., Kaspar, B., Stein, S.A. and Gage, F.H. (2001). Progenitor cells from human brain after death. *Nature*, 411: 42-43.

5. Magavi, S.S., Leavitt, B.R. and Macklis, J.D. (2000). Induction of neurogenesis in the necortex of adult mice. *Nature*, 405: 951-955.

CHAPTER 16

Antibody Engineering and Recombinant Monoclonal Antibodies for Development of New Drugs

After a significant respite during the '80s and most of the '90s, the antibody field has made a comeback. Antibodies are finding applications as therapeutics, as drug delivery vehicles, in diagnostics and imaging, and in drug discovery research for both screening and validation of targets. Among 113 currently approved biotech products currently in the market, monoclonal antibodies form an extremely exciting and emerging business area, with 10 therapeutic antibodies and 5 diagnostic products in the market. Additionally, there are about 75 antibodies currently in clinical trials, constituting nearly 20 per cent of all biotech drugs in development.

The need to overcome the immunogenicity problem of rodent antibodies in clinical practise has resulted in a plethora of strategies to isolate human antibodies. If human antibodies are to be used, then one would like to understand the basis by which different isotypes interact with host effector systems, and, if possible, improve on nature by engineering in desirable modifications.

Humanization of Potential Therapeutic Antibodies

The original humanization strategy described by Winter (1) exploited knowledge of the solved crystal structure with grafting of rodent complementary determining regions (CDRs) into the defined human frameworks, and judicious mutations in critical framework residues (Fig. 16.1).

In order to humanise successfully many other rat and mouse antibodies we adopted a best-fit strategy whereby we selected the most homologous human framework sequence we could find in the databases, and reshaped to that (2, 3, 4). The detailed arguments for and against this strategy have been reviewed in several times.

Defining the Structural Basis of Human Antibody Effector Function

There is still uncertainty about which effector mechanisms determine antibody-mediated cell lysis *in vivo*. *In vitro* readouts such

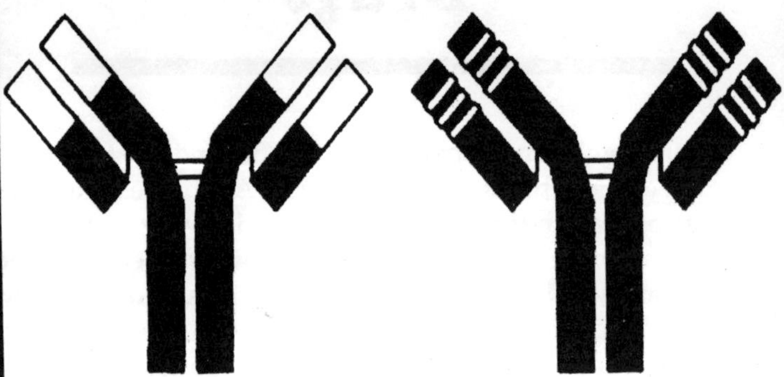

FIGURE 16.1: Schematic Representation of Humanised Antibodies Chimeric (left) and Fully Reshaped (right). In the case of the chimeric antibody the rodent heavy (V_H) and Light chain (V_l) variable regions (white) are attached to human constant regions (black). After full reshaping the four framework regions within each V region are humanised leaving only the six complementarity determining regions (CDR) three in the heavy chain and three in the light chain (white).

as Antibody Dependent Cell-mediated cytotoxicity (ADCC) or complement activation have proven useful in defining differences between isotypes, and in screening of improved antibodies. Because antibodies to the abundant lymphocyte antigen CDw52 (CAMPA TH-I) exhibit potent *in vitro* and *in vivo* lytic potential (1) they have served as the gold standard by which all modifications or mutations could be compared. Each human IgG has 3 homologous constant-region domains (CHI, CH2 and CH3) and a hinge region between CHI and CH2 whose size varies between the isotypes. Some scientists are using matched sets of human antibodies to look for functional differences between the isotypes (5).

By using domain-switch antibodies (6, 7, 8) it can be shown that the differential ability of the isotypes to activate complement depends largely on the carboxy-terminal half of the CH2 domain. Scientist has also shown that this half of the CH2 domain is critical to ADCC through the FcRIII receptor. The binding sites for FcRI and FcRII have both been shown to involve residues in the hinge-link region and the C-terminal half of the CH2 domain. Scientist discovered an interesting polymorphism in human ADCC effector function, whereby some individuals can use all IgG isotypes, while others perform poorly with all the isotypes except for IgG 1 (6).

It is known that to achieve efficient monoclonal antibody-mediated killing, a high antigen-density is advantageous, presumably by approximating sufficient Ig effector domains together. With the knowledge that the CH2 and hinge regions have an important role in effector functions, a series of multiple-domain antibodies that contain extra CH2 and hinge regions have been created (9) and are being investigated for any changes in effector potency (Fig. 16.2).

None of the in tandem series of CAMPA TH-1 antibodies demonstrated better complement lysis than the parent, while the CHl-hinge-CH2-CH2-CH3 form actually lost activity. But an alternative approach providing extra domains in parallel has recently been described by Shopes (10) through creation of dimmers by engineering a cysteine into the H-chain of a chimeric Ig at position 444. The new disulphide bonds were able to link pairs of Ig tail to tail to form covalent dimmers. These novel antibodies were found to have enhanced lytic ability with heterologous complement. Such a dimeric construct has been created for CAMPATH-IH (9), and

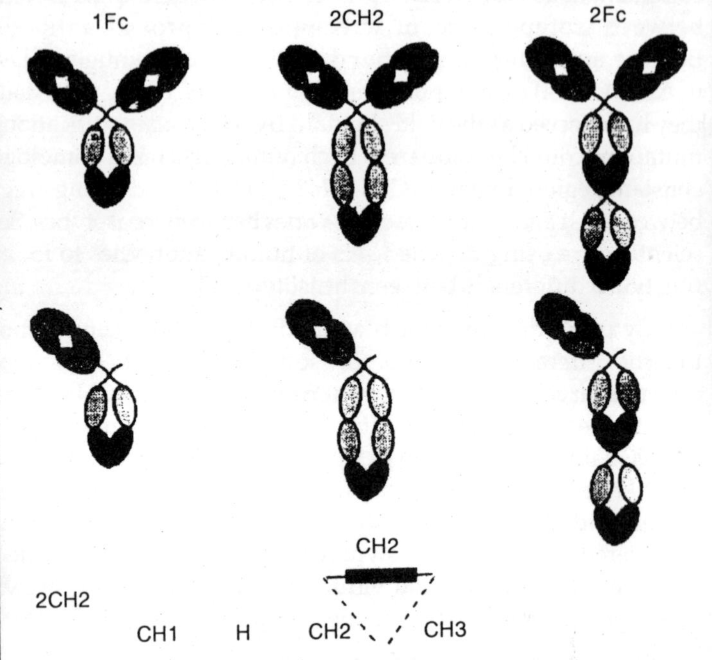

FIGURE 16.2: H-chain Constant Region Domain Duplications

although no more efficient than the monomer for lysis (with homologous complement) of cells expressing high levels of the CAMPATH antigen, it was very efficient at lysing low antigen expressing CCRF-CEM cells, where the parental form (CAMPATH-IH) was non-lytic. It is possible that they may also have enhanced capacity for ADCC. Insufficient information exists yet on potency in ADCC, or performance *in vivo*.

Improving the Performance of a Humanised CD3 Antibody

Antibodies to the CD3 epsilon signalling molecule of the T-cell receptor complex have proven powerful immunosuppressants. OKT3 is widely used for the reversal of allograft rejection episodes. CD3 mAbs like OKT3 could be used more widely were it not for immunogenicity and the toxicity arising from massive cytokine release on first dose administration. Scienfist has taken rat anti-human CD3 antibody (YTH 12.5) and has engineered it to try to address some of the specific (*e.g.* cytokine release) and more general (*e.g.* antigenic modulation without cell destruction) issues that affect therapeutic antibodies. We have produced a humanised version with affinity comparable to the parent (11), and have sought two mutually exclusive directions for antibody improvement. The first was to derive non-lytic, blocking, and non-activating forms that would have efficacy without the side effects of OKT3. The second was to produce more lytic forms that might be better able to kill T-cells thus limiting the extent of cytokine release.

In order to find a form that might block TCR signalling but avoid cytokine release, scientist examined the mitogenicity of a series of isotype-matched variants (12). Scientist surprise all forms (IgGs, IgA and IgE) were mitogenic although IgG2 was less effective. To reduce FcR binding in a hIgG1 form, a mutation was introduced into Asn to convert it to Ala; this destroys the carbohydrate attachment site and results in the synthesis of an, aglycosylated IgG1 heavy chain. This mutant was non-mitogenic *in vitro*, yet powerful at inhibiting T-cell stimulation by antigen.

Rapid antigenic modulation by antibody is a known contributing factor limiting the lysis of cells by antibody and complement. In the past we obtained univalent forms of antibodies from somatic hybrids secreting two light chains, and had shown (13, 14) that such antibodies were better able to activate complement *in vitro*, were still immunosuppressive *in vivo*, and yet surprisingly did not cause cytokine release in the small series studied (10 patients) (14, 15). Given these encouraging preliminary results, Scientist sought to create univalent antibodies by a genetic engineering route.

Scientist derived a truncated H-chain (lacking the VH and CHI domains) as the second C antibody arm, and transfected this into the humanised parental transfectoma (11). While the parental form could not activate complement, the purified univalent antibody was found to be competent. Further analysis of univalent forms of other isotypes revealed that a univalent IgG3 form was even more lytic.

This analysis demonstrates that univalent antibodies with improved complement lytic potency can be generated through relatively simple protein engineering procedures.

References

1. Reichmann, L., Clark, M., Waldmann, H. and Winter, G. (1988). Reshaping human antibodies for therapy. *Nature*, 332: 323-327.
2. Gorman, S.D., Clark, M.R., Routledge, E.G., Cobbold, S.P. & Waldmann, H. (1991). Reshaping a therapeutic CD4 antibody. *Proc. Natl. Acad. Sci.*, 88: 4181-4185.
3. Sims, M.J., Hassal, D.G., Brett, S., Rowan, W., Lockyer, M.J., Angel, A., Lewis, A.P., Hale, G., Waldmann, H. & Crowe, J.S. (1993). A Humanized CD18 Antibody Can Block Function Without Cell Destruction. *The Journal of Immunology*, 51: 2296-2308.
4. Routledge, E.G., Gorman, S.D. & Clark, M. (1993). Reshaping antibodies for therapy. In: *Protein Engineering of Antibody Molecules for Prophylactic and Therapeutic Applications in Man* (Edited by Mike Clark, Cambridge). Academic Titles.
5. Bruggemann, M., Williams, G.T., Bindon C.I., *et al.* (1987). Comparison of the effector function of human immunoglobulins using a matched set of chimeric antibodies. *J. Exp. Med.*, 166: 1351-1361.
6. Greenwood, J., Clark, M. & Waldmann, H. (1993). Structural motifs involved in human IgG antibody effector functions. *Eur. J. of Immunol.*, 23: 1098-1104.
7. Greenwood, J. & Clark, M. (1993). Effector functions of matched sets of recombinant human IgG subclass antibodies. In: *Protein Engineering of Antibody Molecules for Prophylactic and Therapeutic Applications in Man* (Edited by Mike Clark, Cambridge), pp. 85-100, Academic Titles.
8. Morrison, S.L., Caufield, S.M. and Mi-Hua, Tao (1993). Complement activation and Fc receptor binding by Iga. In: *Protein Engineering of Antibody Molecules for Prophylactic and Therapeutic Applications in Man*. Ed M. Clarkp, 101-115, Academic Titles.
9. Greenwood, J., Gorman, S.D., Routledge, E.G., Lloyd, I.S. & Waldmann, H. (1995). Engineering multiple domain forms of the therapeutic antibody CAMPATH-IH: Effects on complement lysis (Personal communication).
10. Shopes, B. (1992). A genetically engineered human IgG mutant with enhanced cytolytic activity. *J. Immunol.*, 148(9): 2918-2922.

recombinant proteins obtained by genetic engineering are in the medical therapeutic fields *(e.g.,* production of recombinant vaccines, and therapeutic proteins for human diseases), and medical diagnosis *(e.g.,* antigen engineering for poly- and monoclonal antibody production used in disease testing) (2). Such therapeutic proteins are interferons, cytokinase (*e.g.*, rG-CSF, rGM-CSF, rIntrlukins), enzymes (rDNase, rGlucocerebrocisidese, rtPA), clotting factors (rFactor IX, rFactor VII), Monoclonal antibodies (Mabs), anticoagulant (rHirudin) and hormones (r EPO, rFSH, rhGH, rTSH, rInsulin, rGlucagon).

Besides producing valuable proteins for practical applications, the production of proteins using recombinant technology offers unprecedented possibilities in the basic research of, protein function, structure, inter-action, turnover, domain shuffling, and many other areas, which could ultimately lead to the development of novel protein applications. Most proteins are expressed in infinitesimal amounts in their native cells and tissues, and it is only by recombinant techniques that it is possible to produce amounts great enough for basic research or for practical uses. Therefore, the expression of engineered proteins in efficient heterologous protein expression system is integral to the production, and purification of many proteins of interest. Moreover, with the vast amounts of predicted protein sequences being generated by genomic research, the application of protein engineering will most certainly be used to better characterize many unknown protein functions, interactions, cellular locations and potential practical uses.

Production Systems for Recombinant Proteins

Although much of recombinant protein engineering is performed *in vitro*, the actual protein synthesis usually utilizes living prokaryotic or eukaryotic cells. Proteins produced *in vivo* can be expressed transiently, constitutively or by induction, with the last two requiring cell lines which stably maintain the genetic material coding for the protein. Another means consist of using live bioreactors, *i.e.*, live transgenic plants and animals, as recombinant protein production systems. The choice of production system depends on many factors including the original source of the protein and codon usage (*e.g.*, prokaryotic, mammalian, plant), post translational processing (*e.g.*, phosphorylation, proteolytic processing, glycosylation, acylation), its future use (*e.g.*, human therapy, plant pest control) and economic factors (3), However, production of any protein is a complex multistep cellular process involving gene transcription, translation, protein processing and localization. Thus, the expression of a recombinant protein in a heterologous host cell or organism is often problematic. For example, protein expression levels can be low, or the purified protein may be insoluble or unstable. And although, certain precautions can be taken *(e.g.,* altering codon usage to match the host's cells), often trial and error is the only real method of operation.

Bacterial Expression Utilizing *E. Coli*

Escherichia coli (*E. coli*) has long been the primary prokaryotic host for heterologous protein expression, therefore there are much informations and technologies available regarding this system with many different proteins (4, 5). The advantages of *E. coli* include its relatively easy, rapid and inexpensive methods of growth, transformation and maintenance. Furthermore, most of the biochemical pathways of *E. coli* are understood in great detail, and its entire genome has been sequenced. Foreign proteins can be produced in *E. coli* in large amounts (5-50 per cent of total protein). Nevertheless, prokaryotic cells such as *E. coli* are unable to perform some post-translational modifications, which occur in eukaryotic cells *(e.g.,* glycosylation, phosphorylation and disulfidebond formation), and which may be crucial for a foreign protein to obtain an active form. The expression and accumulation of a foreign protein in *E. coli* may also cause aggregates of the protein to form (6, 7). Sometimes the protein in these inclusion bodies can be refolded *in vitro* to produce functional protein, but this is not always possible and renaturation can be expensive and time consuming. Furthermore, proteolytic degradation of heterologous protein expression may be a potential obstacle (8). Even though *E. coli* may not be useful for all foreign protein production, it has been successfully utilized to produce many functional human proteins such as human growth hormone, proinsulin, interferon-gamma and antibody fragments (9).

Expression Systems

Various *E. coli* expression systems are available commercially and in the public domain, which is shared within the scientific community. Each system offers different benefits for protein expression, detection, and purification, and should be considered according to the specific criteria and requirements each protein poses. The expression unit or cassette in which the foreign protein coding region will be cloned into should consist of a strong promoter (*e.g.*, T7, trc, lac, tac, PL, PR, phoA, ara, xapA, cad, recA), ribosomal binding site(s), and, an efficient transcription terminator (5). Tightly controlled transcription coupled with a strong and rapid transcription inducer (*e.g.*, IPTG, tryptophan, temperature, phosphatase starvation, rabinose, xanthosine, pH, nalidixic acid) are crucial for high protein expression. Other factors to be considered include convenient multiple cloning sites, appropriate codon usage, and plasmid copy number. Usually, high protein expression levels are desirable, but in cases where the protein may form insoluble inclusion bodies, or may be toxic to the bacterial host, lower and slower expression may be preferred. The ideal promoter for expression directs efficient transcription to allow high level production, and is tightly regulated to minimize the metabolic burden and toxic effects of a foreign protein. Regulatable promoters are used to drive foreign protein expression to avoid the selection of non-expressing mutant cells during the cell growth phase. Promoters such as T3, SP6 and T7 are widely used and efficient promoters derived from *E. coli* bacteriophages. The T7 RNA polymerase is very specific for its own promoter, and can transcribe RNA templates approximately five times faster than the *E. coli* RNA polymerase. The gene coding for T7 RNA polymerase is either lysogenic or it is transfected into the cell by the bacteriophage CE6. In DE3 *E. coli* cells the T7 RNA polymerase gene is under the control of the *LacUV5* promoter, which is inducible by IPTG. The addition of IPTG to a culture of DE3 cells will induce the transcription of T7 RNA polymerase, which in turn transcribes any gene under the control of the T7 promoter. However, the basal level of T7 RNA polymerase activity will promote some transcription of the target gene in non-induced cells. More strict control mechanisms have been engineered to depress basal T7 RNA polymerase expression. One method is based on the addition of a regulatory *lacl* gene, which codes for a strong repressor of the *LacUV5* promoter. Very low basal expression levels of target gene can be reduced even more by adding T7 lysozyme, yet high level expression can be achieved upon induction with IPTG. Moreover, the T7*lacO* expression vectors pBAT, pHAT and pRAT have been reported to be suitable for expression of toxic proteins in *E. coli* (10). In these vectors tight control is achieved by centering the *lac* operator 14 base pairs downstream from the major RNA transcription start point.

Solubility

The majority of foreign proteins produced in *E. coli* are cytosolic, but as mentioned above some proteins accumulate as aggregates called inclusion bodies. In these aggregates only a small fraction of the protein is folded correctly, and the rest is in a denatured and usually non-functional form (11). The probability of any heterologous protein forming inclusion bodies correlates greatly with its charge average and turn forming residue fraction, whereas hydrophilicity and total number of residues do not appear to correlate with inclusion body formation (12).

Inclusion bodies may consist of not only the foreign protein, but also of some host components such as T7 RNA polymerase, membrane components, 16S and 23S RNA and even plasmid DNA. In some cases the formation of inclusion bodies can be advantageous, since the expressed protein can be purified simply by washing and pelleting the aggregated bodies (13). However, often the aggregation of the protein is detrimental, therefore expression conditions must be optimized so that the possibility of producing soluble protein is increased. The maximized solubility of a protein can be achieved by optimizing several factors such as the expression temperature, *E.coli* strain used, pH of the growth medium, fusion partner the protein is fused with, rate and level of expression and co-expression with chaperones and foldases (14). For example, fusions to ZZ (two domains derived from staphylococcal protein A) and thioredoxin have been reported to increase the solubility of insulin-like growth factor land cytokines (15). Chaperone proteins mediate both the folding and rehabilitation of proteins. The most extensively studied chaperons/foldases in *E. coli* are GroEL/GroES, which have been reported to assist in folding proteins into active forms (16). Moreover, co-overproduction of thioredoxin has been reported to increase the solubility of insulin-like growth factor I as well as other vertebrate proteins expressed in *E. coli.* However, even if co-overexpression of chaperons/foldases *(e.g.,* GroES, GroEL, DnaK) is likely to be useful for some proteins, it is unlikely to provide a universal solution to the problem of inclusion formation. Other factors affecting protein solubility include regulation of the expression vector and bacterial cell lysis methods. Protein inclusion bodies are usually solubilized using urea or guanidine hydrocloride (Gdn-HCl). After denaturation the protein must be renatured under conditions that favor their proper folding and native functions. Conditions that must be considered when trying to refold a denatured protein involve optimizing the renaturation temperature (usually around 10°C), redox conditions, protein concentration, and addition of solubilizing additives such as polyethylene glycol.

Soluble and active proteins have also been obtained with treatment with N dodecanoyl-sarcosinate, (17).

Secretion

Secretion of foreign proteins to the medium can greatly facilitate their purification.

However, secretion of a protein to the medium by Gram-negative bacteria, such as *E. coli*, requires translocation of the protein through the bacterial cell wall consisting of inner and outer membrane bilayers surrounding the penplasmic space. Only a limited number of *E. coli* strains are capable of secreting proteins from the cell (reviewed in Pugsley, 1993). Nevertheless, some genetically modified proteins with inserted secretion sequence signals have been successfully secreted into the media (18). More importantly, *E. coli* is capable of secreting genetically altered proteins into the periplasm, which may represent 20-40 per cent of the total cellular volume. With this strategy the target protein can be separated from the cytoplasmic proteins and accumulating a more oxidizing environment where disulfide-bond formation can occur. Secretion into the enplasmic space has been successfully utilized in large scale production of biologically active antibody fragments.

Yeast (*Saccharomyces cerevisiae*)

Saccharomyces cerevisiae (bakers and brewers yeast) is generally considered as a safe organism for the production of foreign proteins, since it has been used in food production for thousands of years. This unicellular eukaryote has been extensively studied at the biochemical, molecular and genomic levels, and its entire genome has been recently sequenced (19). Like *E. coli*, yeast grows rapidly in relatively inexpensive and simple media, is easy to transform, and maintain. But unlike *E. coli*, yeast is an eukaryotic cell, and therefore expresses and processes proteins more similarly to higher eukaryotes. The secretory pathway of yeast closely resembles that of mammalian cells, thus yeast is capable of many post translational modifications such as proteolytic processing, disulfide bond formation, and glycosylation. Thus, yeast offers a eukaryotic protein production system that can retain the foreign protein intracellularly or the product can be secreted to the medium if fused to a carrier peptide. However, *S. cerevisiae* is unable to perform certain complex eukaryotic post-translational modifications such as prolylhydroxylation and amidation. In addition, the glycosylation of yeast can differ from that of higher eukaryotes. Nevertheless, many foreign proteins have been produced on a large scale using *S. cerevisiae,* including human serum albumin, the hepatitis B viral surface antigen, insuling and hirudin (20).

Episomal Vectors and Chromosomal Integration

Recombinant DNA which encodes foreign proteins can be expressed in *S. cerevisiae* as an episomal plasmid or integrated into its genome. Extra-chromosomal replicons are based either on plasmids containing autonomously replicating sequences, or on the native 2μ circle of *S. cerevisiae.* Most yeast expression vectors have been constructed from the multi-copy 2μ plasmid, which has also been engineered to replicate and be selectable in both *E. coli* and reported to increase transcriptional activity (21), as well as regulate the overproduction of the GAL4 protein.

Secretion of Heterologous Proteins

S. cerevisiae is capable of secreting heterologous proteins, but most of them have to be fused to an appropriate pre-pro-leader. These carriers are relatively short amino acid sequences and include pre-pro-leaders from such proteins as _-factor, killer-toxin, bar protease, gp3 7, and Hsp 150. The carrier peptide may have a crucial role in the transport process from the ER to the Golgi, which has been suggested to be receptor-mediated. The carrier may thus provide a positive secretion signal for the capture of fusion protein into vesicle budding sites at the ER membrane (22). The carrier may also assist the fusion partner to acquire a secretion-competent conformation. Some proteins can be externalized in *S. cerevisiae* without a carrier. Human lipo-cortin-1 was first expressed as a fusion with the α factor pre-pro-region but only 10 per cent of the protein was secreted (23). An expression system utilizing the inunilase signal peptide increased secreted lipocortin-1 5-fold, resulting up to 95 per cent of the protein to be secreted into the medium (23). Furthermore, fed-batch fermentation of the heterologous protein produced 2.1 g/l, representing more than 80 per cent of the total extracellular protein (23). Also, it has been observed that culture growth conditions can affect protein secretion. For example, B-galactosidase, which is normally refractile to secretion, is secreted from yeast grown in a rich medium. B-galactosidase secretion could be further increased by elevated growth temperatures.

Yeast Secretory Proteins as Carriers

In *S. cerevisiae* the most commonly used carrier is the pre-pro-region of the factor. The pre-sequence (signal sequence) is cleaved upon translocation into the ER and the pro- region is cleaved by the Kex2 protease in the Golgi compartment. However, the mechanisms which the pre-pro-region uses to confer secretion competence to the

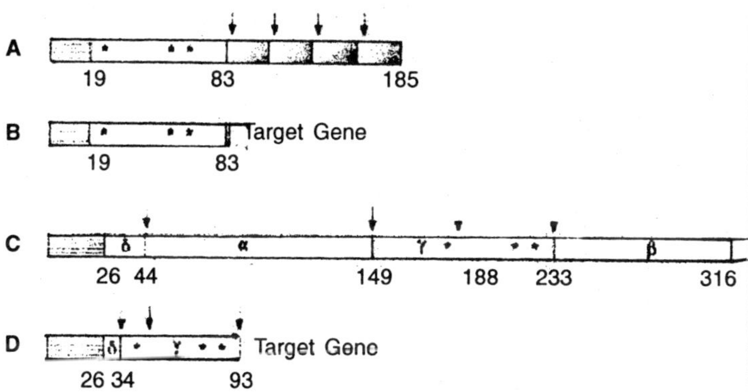

FIGURE 17.1: A Schematic Presentation of Primary Translation Products of *S. cerevisiae*. A: Pre-pro-region of α factor used as a carrier, B: Killer toxin, C: pre-pro-region of killer toxin used as a carrier, D: Pre-pro-killer toxin carrier comprises killer toxin residues 1-34, which are joined by alanine to the gamma-region residues 177-233. The Kex2 cleavage and N-glycosylation sites are indicated by arrows and asterisks, respectively. The signal sequence is marked by a horizontally striped area and the repetitive region of α factor is colored gray.

fusion partners as well as its structure, are not known. Synthetic leaders have also been used as carriers. Interestingly, it appears that three N-linked oligosaccharide chains are necessary for secretion competence of the factor pre-pro-leader, whereas synthetic pre-pro-leaders lacking the consensus N-glycosylation sites confers secretion competence of correctly folded insulin precursors. Another polypeptide used as a carrier in yeast is derived from the killer toxin. The K1 killer toxin is a heterodimer of two protein subunits (α and β), maturated from the 316 residue pre-pro-.toxin. As in the pre-pro-region factor, the signal sequence of the pre-pro-toxin is cleaved upon translocation into the ER and the pro-region is subsequently cleaved by the Kex2 protease in the Golgi compartment. The ability of different fragments of the killer toxin pre-pro-region to confer secretion competence for heterologous protein was studied by fusing β-lactamase to various fragments of pre-pro-toxin.

The Secretion Pathway of *S. cerevisiae*

The secretory pathway in eukaryotic cells is essential for posttranslational processing, targeting and transporting proteins to intra- and extracellular membranes and for proteins destined for export out of the cell. The secretory pathway of yeast is depicted in Figure 17.2. It consists of several membrane-bound compartments and vesicle-trafficing systems between these compartments. Protein secretion in yeast has been studied using, temperature-sensitive secretion *(sec)* mutants, in which the transport of proteins can be reversibly blocked in distinct compartments. Secretory proteins have a signal peptide, which is an endoplasmic reticulum (ER) targeting sequence present usually at their Nterminus, which allows the protein to enter the ER. Most posttranslational, modifications, such as the initiation of glycosylation, disulfide bond formation and protein folding occur in the ER. Transport to the next compartment, the *cis* Golgi, occurs by vesicular transport, which is also the way proteins are transported through the Golgi (intra-Golgi) to the *trans* Golgi network (TGN). Transport, docking, and fusion of transport vesicles are regulated by proteins generally referred to as SNAREs (reviewed by Gerst, 1999). The anterograde and/or retrograde membrane traffic between the ER and Golgi occurs in vesicles coated with COPI and COPII proteins (25). In the TGN proteins are sorted into distinct vesicles, which are estined to the plasma membrane or to vacuoles (26). The sorting to vacuoles occurs *via* a late endosome-

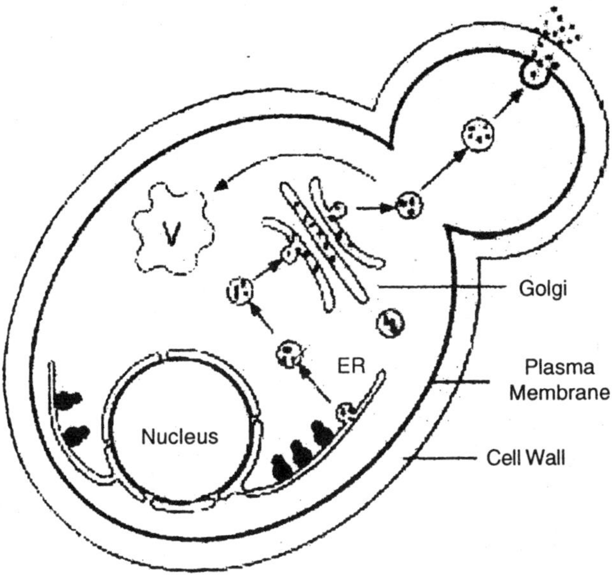

FIGURE 17.2: A Schematic Presentation of the Secretory Route of Yeast *S. cerevisiae.* The nascent secretory proteins are translocated into the lumen of the endoplasmic reticulum (ER), from where they are transported by carrier vesicles *via* the, Golgi to the vacuole, the plasma membrane, the cell wall or to the growth medium. Reproduction from Saris (1998) with permission.

like prevacuolar compartment. The ER signal sequence consists of a short hydrophobic peptide with hydrophilic residues at both ends Polypeptides are translocated into the lumen of the ER usually cotranslationally, although some proteins translocate posttranslationally. During cotranslational translocation, the signal sequence of a nascent polypeptide is first recognized by the signal recognition particle (SRP) (27). After binding to the SRP, translation is arrested until the complex is bound to the ER membrane *via* the SRP receptor. The translocation of proteins occurs through translocation channels containing hetero-trimeric complexes of the Sec61 protein. The signal peptides of proteins which translocate posttranslationally are less hydrophobic and are thus independent

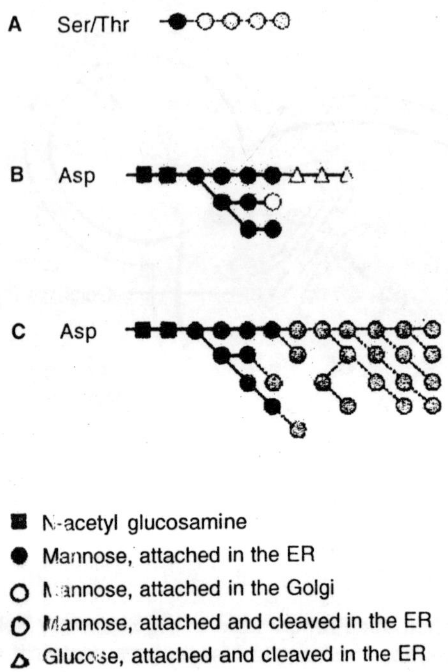

FIGURE 17.3: Carbohydrate Structures of *S. cerevisiae* glycoproteins. A: The first mannose of an o-linked oligosaccharide is attached to a serine (Ser) or threonine (Thr) residue in the ER and the chain is elongated up to pentamannosides in the Golgi compartment, B: An N-acetallucosamine is attached to an asparagine (Asp) residue to from the core structure of N-linked oligosaccharide in the ER and (C) the outer chains are elongated in the Golgi. The length of the outer chain varies from 2 to 15 mannose residues.

of SRP. Posttranslational translocation requires a complex of Sec62, Sec63, Sec71 and Sec72 proteins in addition to the Sec61 translocon channel. The BiP chaperone has a critical role in translocation. It binds to the translocating polypeptide, acting as a molecular ratchet thus preventing the backsliding of the protein (28).

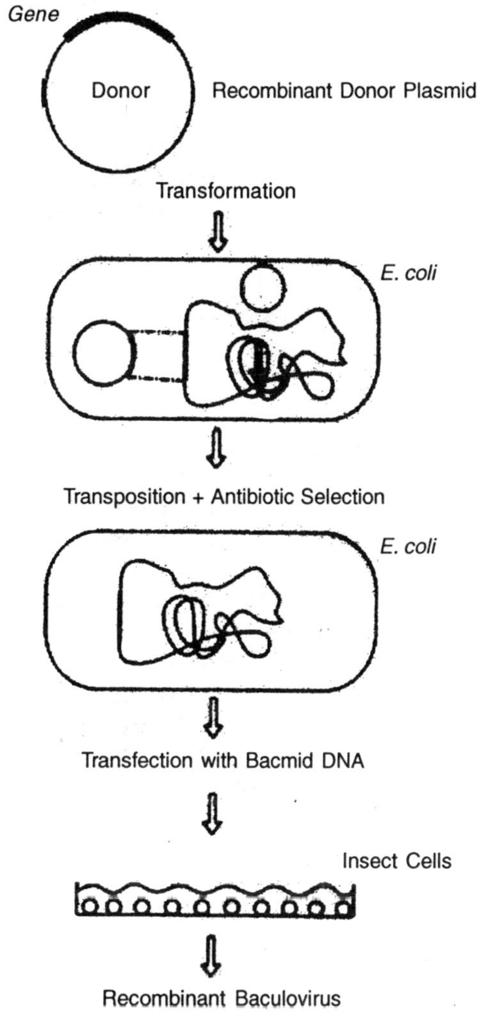

FIGURE 17.4: Schematic Outline of the Generation of Recombinant Baculovirus with a Bac-to-Bac Expression System. A donor vector carrying the gene of interest flanked by a Tn7-element is transformed to *E. coli.* The Tn7 element can integrate into the attTn7 target site in the presence of transposition proteins provided by a helper plasmid. Recombinant bacmids are selected using -their antibiotic resistance and recombinant bacmid DNA is used to transfect insect cells.

The ER is the main location where secretory proteins fold and it contains several folding enzymes and chaperone proteins essential for proper protein folding and transport. The lumen of the ER is an oxidizing environment and contains high levels of calcium, which provides proper conditions for chaperones and disulfide bond formation. Signal peptidase and glycosyltransferase complexes are functionally associated, and signal sequence cleavage and glycosylation, together with protein folding occur cotranslationally in the ER. In yeast cells, proteins are glycosylated with N-linked and O-linked glycans. Glycosylation is assumed to promote correct folding, protect against proteolysis and thermal denaturation, as well as to egulate intracellular trafficking. In O-linked oligosaccharides, the first mannose residue is attached to a serine or threonine in the ER, which is unlike mammalian cells where mucin-type O-glycosylation is initiated in the Golgi by adding an N-acetyl-galactosamine to the fully folded protein. O-linked oligosaccharide chains in yeast can be elongated up to 5 mannoses in the Golgi whereas O-glycans in mammalian cells are elongated by adding mannose, galactose, Nacetyl glucosamine, fucose, sialylate residues and/or polylactosamine-extensions (29). N-glycosylation of secreted glycoproteins in yeast is initiated in the ER. In yeast, the core oligosaccharide consisting of two N-acetyl glucosamine, nine mannose residues and three glucose residues is similar to that of higher eukaryotes. Unlike mammalian cells, the mannose residues are not replaced by other sugars (N-acetyl glucosamine, galactose, fucose and sialic acid) in the Golgi, but the outer chains are elongated by mannose residues only.

Optimizing Expression

The genetic background of both natural and recombinant yeast strains have been found to affect the quantity and structure of heterologous proteins.

Because different genetic backgrounds can influence transcription and translation efficiencies, the secretory pathway, protein quality, plasmid stability and plasmid copy number, it may be necessary to screen a number of different host strains with varying genetic backgrounds when optimizing heterologous protein expression in yeast. Some genetic background considerations that may aid in foreign protein production in yeast include: the use of proteasedeficient strains, which can decrease heterologous protein degradation thus increasing yields, and the 'use of strains lacking hyperglycosylation of N-linked sites. However, these strains usually grow slower than normal strains, but there, are also yeast strains that require relatively few generations to obtain high production yields. An N-terminus sequence of human interleukin α could be utilized as an enhancer for heterologous protein expression in the way as has been reported for two human growth hormones (30). And, as in *E. coli,* the coexpression of chaperones have been reported to assist in the proper folding and secretion of foreign proteins in *S. cerevisiae.* Furthermore, the overexpression of disulfide isomerase (PDI) resulted in a 10-fold increase in secreted human platelet-derived growth factor, a four fold increase in acid phosphatase, a two to eight fold increase for five single chain antibody fragments (31), and a 15 to 24-fold increase in antistasin.

Insect Cells (Baculovirus System)

The baculovirus expression system (BVS) is commonly used to express heterologous proteins in insect cells. Since insect cells are eukaryotic, proteins expressed in them will be posttranslationally modified in a manner similar to that of mammalian cells. Insect cells can be grown as suspension cultures, which permits the use of large-scale bioreactors for easier production scale-up. Furthermore, unlike mammalian cell lines insects cells do not require CO_2-incubators.The most commonly used baculovirus system utilized *Autographa californica* Multiple Nuclear Polyhedrosis virus (AcMNPV) in a cell line derived from Lepidopteran *Spodoptera frugiperda* ovarian cells (Sf9). The AcMNPV's genome is a double-stranded, circular DNA, approximately 130 kilobases in length, and has been fully sequenced. The production systems are commonly regulated by strong promoters like polyhedrin and p10 but also immediate early promoters (for example *iel)* have been utilized. Latter expression systems gave a continuous and stable expression of human glycoprotein in both infected and transformed Lepidopteran cells (32). As an alternative to baculovirus expression systems, an expression cassette for continuous protein expression by transformed insect have also been developed (33). The system utilizes the promoter of the silkmoth cytoplasmic actin gene, the iel transactivator gene and the HR3 enhancer region of *Bombyx mori* MNPV to stimulate gene expression. Levels of produced proteins in this system are comparable to the ones produced in BVS.

Systems Utilizing Polyhedrin and p10

In general, wild type baculoviruses exhibit lytic and occluded life cycles, producing extra cellular and occlusion derived virus (ODV), respectively. ODV is embedded in proteinaceous viral occlusions called polyhedra. Polyhedrin, a 29 kD protein, is the major component of polyhedra, which in turn are crystalline occlusion bodies visible in the nuclei of infected cells by light microscopy. The expression of viral genes is regulated in a successive cascade consisting of 4 distinguishable phases: early, delayed early, late and very late (34). During the very late phase of viral replication two very abundant mRNAs are produced, one of which codes for the polyhedrin protein and other codes for the p10 protein (10 kDa). The p10 polypeptide is involved in the formation of fibrillar structures found both in the nucleus and in the cytoplasm of baculovirus infected cells. The role of polyhedra is to protect occluded baculoviruses after the death of infected insects, and its presence is essential for the maintenance of the virus in nature. However, viral propagation in cell cultures is based on virions which bud from infected cells, not on ODV, Thus, baculovirus expression vectors have been engineered in which the *polyhedrin* and *p10* coding regions are deleted, but their strong promoters are retained to express foreign proteins in large amounts in the late and very late phases of infection. In the baculovirus expression system utilizing the *p10* promoter, the sequence encoding the p10 protein as well as the entire polyhedrin locus, including its promoter, have been deleted (35). The remaining *p10* promoter is used to express recombinant protein sequences. In this way, expression of both the native polyhedrin and p10 proteins are abolished, which reduces background problems caused by the expression of large amounts of very late native proteins while increasing the expression of foreign recombinant proteins.

Furthermore, the *p10* promoter is activated earlier in the infection cycle than the *polyhedrin* promoter (36). The absence of the p10 protein results in delayed cell lysis, and thereby an extended period of recombinant protein synthesis. The yields of two reporter enzymes, juvenile hormone esterase and β-galactosidase were higher under the *p10* promoter compared to *polyhedrin* controlled expression (36).

Recombination

In baculovirus expression systems the insertion of genes coding for foreign proteins can be accomplished by homologous recombination, site-specific transposition (Bac-to-Bac) or insertion directly into the viral genome *in vitro*. In homologous recombination, the gene of interest is cloned into a transfer vector containing a baculovirus promoter flanked by baculovirus DNA derived from the polyhedrin gene. After transfection into insect,. cells, the gene is inserted into the genome of the parent virus by homologous recombination, at a rate of approximately 0.1 to 1 per cent. Recombinants are identified by their altered plaque morphology, which appears as 'occlusion minus' plaques. A higher rate of recombination can be achieved when the parent virus genome is linearized at site(s) near the target site of foreign gene insertion Kitts and Possee (1993)(37) reported recombination rates approaching 100 per cent when they used linearized viral DNA that is missing an essential portion of the baculovirus genome downstream from the polyhedrin locus. Nevertheless, by this method it can take more than a month to purify the plaques, and confirm the desired recombinants. A faster, method to generate recombinant baculovirus can be achieved by utilizing baculovirus. Ac-omega, which contains an unique restriction site downstream of the polyhedrin promoter. By this method recombinant viruses were obtained 8 days posttransfection and according to PCR analysis the non-recombinant background was 25 fold lower than that of the recombinant viral DNA. Another method utilizing site-specific transposition is also relatively fast (7-10 days) because plaque purification or virus amplification are not needed. In this method, the foreign gene is cloned into a baculovirus shuttle vector (bacmid) that can replicate in *E. coli,* but can also infect susceptible lepidopteran insect cells. Bacmid is a recombinant virus that contains a mini-F replicon, a kanamycin resistance marker, and attTn7, the target site for the bacterial transposon Tn7 (38). Expression cassettes comprising a baculovirus promoter driving expression of a foreign gene that is flanked by the left and right ends of Tn7, can transpose to the target bacmid in *E. coli* when Tn7 transposition functions are provided by a helper plasmid.

Optimizing Expression

The density at which cells are infected, and the multiplicity of infection (m.o.i.) greatly affects the expression of heterologous proteins. For instance, when the integral membrane protein bovine rhodpsin was expressed in large amounts, the highest volumetric yields were obtained with an m.o.i. of 0.01 during early to mid-exponential growth (39). For easier purification, and cost saving reasons, it is possible to produce heterologous, proteins in Sf9 cells in serum-free and protein-free media. The cells were gradually adapted to serum-free media in monolayer cultures and reached a doubling time of approximately 25 h, compared with 18 h in serum containing medium. Furthermore, the control of proteolysis in insect cells has a important role when optimizing the yield of recombinant protein (35). Like in *S. cerevisiae,* unwanted mannose residues can be added to secreted glycoproteins and they lack penultimate galactose as well as terminal sialic acid residues. The immediate early promoters (for example *iel*), have been shown to be beneficial for protein production *e.g.*, when highly glycosylated or otherwise modified proteins are to be produced (40).

Mammalian Expression System Utilizing Vaccinia and Alphavirus Vectors

In some cases, mammalian cell systems are the only possible way to produce properly processed and active foreign proteins. Gene transfer into mammalian cells may be performed either by infection with a virus carrying the recombinant gene of interest or by direct transfer of plasmid DNA (41).

Vaccinia Virus Vector

Recombinant vaccinia virus vectors have generally been acknowledged as versatile tools for the expression of foreign genes. Since vaccinia is infectious to man, safety aspects must be taken into consideration, especially when working with large-scale preparations. To circumvent safety problems, an avian host-restricted vaccinia, modified vaccinia Ankara (MVA), can be used (42). Furthermore, MVA does not produce the rapid cytophatic effect accompanied by destruction of the cell monolayer seen with the standard replication strains of vaccinia used. MVA has been shown to efficiently produce foreign proteins in several mammalian cell lines using either the homologous vaccinia promoter, *p11* or a hybrid vaccinia/bacteriophage T7 promoter system (42). In the vaccinia/T7 polymerase hybrid system, the vaccinia virus contains the T7 RNA polymerase gene, which is under the control of an early vaccinia promoter. The foreign gene to be expressed is cloned into a separate expression vector under the control of the *T7* promoter. After the host cells are infected with the vaccinia/T7 virus, the cells are transfected with the expression plasmid. Problems with vaccinia systems include their cytopathic nature, and dependence on efficient transfection rates. Mammalian cell lines can be engineered so that the genes to be transfected are stably integrated into the cell's genome, but then a tightly controlled-inducible promoter must be used. This method is especially advantageous when foreign protein production must be scaled-up. Furthermore, homologous vaccinia promoter systems can be more effective in producing secreted foreign proteins as compared to the heterologous T7 promoter system.

Another vaccinia virus based expression system utilizes defective vaccinia virus lacking the D4R open reading frame, and a complementary cell line providing the D4R gene product (43). Experiments done with human secreted proteins (*i.e.,* factors VII and XI) showed that the defective system produces more secreted proteins than the wild type vaccinia. Surprisingly, recombinant human factor VII was more efficiently produced using the defective vaccinia recombinant under non-complementing conditions (43). This suggests that the persistence of early phase vaccinia replication, combined with a delay in the shutoff of host protein synthesis, can be advantageous for foreign protein production.

Alphavirus Vectors

Semliki Forest (SFV) and Sindbis (SIN) viruses together with Venezuelan equine encephalitis virus are used as vectors for the expression of heterologous proteins in many diverse cells types. Alphavirus replicon vectors are self-replicating RNA molecules which include the genes for nonstructural proteins (Nsps), while lacking the genes of the viral structural proteins. Instead of the structural genes, cloning sites have been engineered to accept foreign genes for expression. The replicons are introduced into host cells by transfection either as RNA, synthesized *in vitro,* or as DNA under the control of an eukaryotic promoter. Iternatively, the recombinant alphavirus RNA can be packaged into viral particles in cells that have been cotransfected with replication competent, but packaging incompetent helper RNA coding for the alphavirus structural proteins. Although, recombination between vector and helper genomes can generate a fully infectious virus, this usually happens at very low frequencies. One way to prevent this recombination is to use conditional mutations to limit the infectivity of any such recombinants (44). In an improved packaging system, the helper virus has been modified so that the structural proteins are expressed in two separate, plasmids. As vaccinia systems, alphavirus infections shuts off the host's own protein synthesis, which makes protein purification easier. Compared to vaccinia, SFV is less cytopathic to the host, and thereby potentially more efficient in foreign protein production. Furthermore, non-pathogenic alphavirus vectors have been developed. For example, a Sindbis virus derivative, which has low host cell pathogenicity due to a single point mutation in Nsp2, demonstrates a persistent infection, while its replication rate is as high as the one of the wild type SIN (45). Although expression of foreign proteins using alphaviruses derived vectors can generate very high yields (up to 25 per cent of total cellular proteins), cloning of large foreign genes into replicons can be problematic. Foreign sequences of about 2 kb are usually stable in SIN vectors, whereas various inserts over 3 kb were rapidly deleted suggesting that the packaging capacity of the virion had been exceeded. Besides tissue and suspension culture applications of alphavirus replicons, *in situ* infections and foreign protein expression have been accomplished in the neurons of rat hippocampal slices. This system has been used to produce β-galactosidase, tissue plasminogen, chloramphenicol acetyl transferase, hemagglutinin and Hepadnavirus proteins. Furthermore, derivatives of alphavirus vectors have been used to direct foreign protein expression in specific cell types in a tissue (46).

Purification Strategies for Recombinant Proteins

Purification is an important step in the production of recombinant proteins. The characteristics of industrial-scale purification schemes, such as conventional chromatography, have a significant impact on the final cost of production. It is often, more efficient to use one of the available tags to 'fish out' the target protein. The purpose for which the protein will be used determines required degree for its purity and authenticity. To purify intracellularly produced proteins the cells are harvested and lysed, which naturally contributes to the complexity of the protein mixture. The advantage of intracellular versus secreted protein is the volume to be handled, *i.e.*, the secreted proteins usually exist diluted in the culture medium. Isolation of a desired protein from the medium follows the general scheme:

1. Concentration by precipitation, ultrafiltration, batch adsorption or partition in an aqueous phase system
2. Enrichment by chromatography or partition
3. High resolution purification: by chromatography and/or immuno adsorption
4. Final concentration.

If fetal calf serum (FCS) is used in cultivation, bovine serum albumin and globulins will be the most abundant proteins in the supernatant. The interaction of albumin especially with hydrophobic proteins represents a significant problem for the effective purification of minor constituents. Even though there are many existing examples as well as heuristics and complex algorithms for suggesting the potential of purification processes, no universal scheme has been developed which could be applied to all proteins. There are a variety of different methods which can be used to purify proteins, but only chromatographic purification methods such as affinity, ion exchange, reversed phase and gel filtration chromatography will be briefly reviewed here.

Conventional Chromatography

Chromatographic methods (size exclusion, ion exchange, reversed phase, hydrophobic interaction and affinity based) can be utilized either in traditional, low pressure or high performance liquid chromatography instrumentation. In addition to liquid-solid chromatography there is liquid-liquid chromatography which is analogous to gas-liquid chromatography (47). There are also many other types of chromatography methods *e.g.*, liquid adsorption chromatography, frontal chromatography, displacement chromatography covalent chromatography and membrane chromatography (48).

Ion Exchange Chromatography

Ion exchange chromatography (IEC) has been the most widely used technique for the isolation and purification of biological macromolecules since the 1950s (49). IEC is able to separate almost any type of charged molecules, from large proteins to small nucleotides and amino acids. The ion exchanger are insoluble solid matrices containing fixed ionogenic groups which bind reversibly to sample molecules (proteins, etc.). Desorption is then brought about by increasing the salt concentration or by altering the pH of the mobile phase. The two major classes of ion exchangers are cation exchangers and anion exchangers, having negatively and positively charged functional groups, respectively. Ion exchange containing diethyl aminoethyl (DEAE) or carboxymethyl (CM) groups are most frequently used. Since the protein is covered by a hydrophilic layer, electrostatic interactions have a major role in the retention of proteins. In addition to size, geometric form as well as hydrophopic and van der Waals interactions affect the separation (50). Nevertheless, the major property which govern the adsorption to an ion exchanger is the net surface charge of the protein. Since surface charge is the result of weak acidic and basic groups on proteins, separation is highly pH-dependent. The optimum pH range for IEC for many proteins is within 1 pH units of the isoelectric point. Many retention models have been examined but the complexity of the adsorption process for a protein to solid surfaces makes it difficult to construct physical models for the interactions (50). Gradient elution with increasing salt concentration is most commonly used in the IEC. The higher the net charge of the protein, the higher the ionic strength needed to bring about desorption. Thus, to optimize selectivity in ion exchange chromatography, the pH of the running buffer is chosen so that sufficiently large net charge differences among the sample components are created.

Reversed Phase Chromatography

Reversed phase chromatography (RPC) can be utilized to separate compounds according to their hydrophobicity. Unlike many other methods RPC is able to separate closely related and structurally disparate substances, even at picomolar levels. In RPC, silica particles covered with chemically-bonded hydrocarbon chains represent the lipophilic phase (C2 to C18), while an aqueous mixture of an organic solvent surrounding the particle represents the hydrophilic phase (51). Depending on the extractive power of the eluent, a greater or lesser part of the sample component will be retained reversibly by the lipid layer of the particles. The partitioning of the sample components between the two phases will depend on their respective solubility characteristics. Less hydrophobic components will end up primarily in the hydrophilic phase while more hydrophobic ones will be found in the lipophilic phase. This can be affected by the addition of an organic solvent which is soluble in the hydrophilic phase. Some commonly used organic solvents, in order of increasing hydrophobicity are methanol, propanol, acetonitrile, and.etrahydrofuran. Separated components can be directly subjected to further analysis such as Edman sequencing or electrospray mass spectrometry. The ability of a stationary phase (lipophilic phase) to discriminate between two components is reflected by the volume between the peak maxima of the corresponding zones after passing through the column. Along with partitioning, mechanism adsorption operates at the interface between the mobile and the stationary phases. Thus, the retention of hydrophobic components will be greatly influenced by the thickness of the lipid layer. AC18 layer is able to accommodate more hydrophobic material than C8 or C2 ones. For hydrophilic components, changing from a C18 to a C2 layer influences the separation very little since only the surface area of the lipid layer is active. The mobile phase can be considered as an aqueous solution of an organic solvent, the type and concentration of which determines the extractive power. Moreover, according to experimental data, components interact with the chromatographic surface in an orientation-specific manner. RPC has been utilized for purification of a variety of proteins and peptides *e.g.*, aprotinin, cytochrome, bovine serum albumin, fibrinogen, insulin and lysosyme (52). Even though some proteins have been reported to maintain their native structure during RPC (*e.g.*, insulin, thyroid-stimulating hormone, growth hormone), in most cases denaturing conditions are required which might limit the use of RPC.

Gel Permeation Chromatography

The principle of gel permeation chromatography (GPC; size exclusion or gel filtration chromatography) is based on molecular volumes. Large molecules are excluded from the matrix, whereas intermediate size molecule can partly enter and only small molecules can freely enter the matrix. The porous three dimensional matrix acts as a steric barrier to solute molecules as they attempt to equilibrate with liquid inside and outside the bead. While purifying the protein GPC can also be used to estimate approximate molecular weights. Furthermore, gel filtration can be used for desalting or buffer changing when the fractionated size of the gel is small (*e.g.*, Bio-Gel 6, Sephadex G-25) allowing the protein to elute in the void volume. The choice of the appropriate column type depends on the molecular size and physical properties of the proteins to be separated. A fraction of the internal volume which is accessible to a solute molecule can be described by a constant Kd, which can be calculated with experimentally determined elution volumes. A column should be chosen so that separations occur in the linear part of the Kd vs. the molecular weight plot (53). However, it is practically impossible to adjust the pH and ionic strength so that the proteins are in an equal state, since at the isoelectric point the shape of globular and polymer coil proteins relieve compact and soft sphere, respectively. Furthermore, the ionic strength of the buffer used may affect the size of the proteins. Experiments with neutral dextrans and charged proteins showed that the effective protein size increases with decreasing ionic strength due to the reduction in electrostatic shielding (54). Thus, although GPC is viewed as size-based separation process, there is considerable evidence for the importance of electrostatic interactions as well. GPC has been used in the renaturation procedure (55, 56). For example heterodimeric platelet-derived growth factor was purified from inclusion bodies after denaturation with Gdn-HCI (55). Renaturation of this growth factor involved folding into an active heterodimeric form during GPC while circumventing aggregation observed when refolding was carried out by dilution.

Affinity Chromatography

Affinity chromatography together with recombinant DNA-technology offers a simple and fast technique to purify proteins to high purity with a single purification step. Fusion can be made on either 'side or both sides of the target gene depending on specific application, but the majority of fusion proteins place the tag at the N-terminus of the protein (57). Genetic manipulation of the protein can be used to form a cleavage site, which helps to remove the affinity tag after purification thereby resulting in an intact protein. Although affinity chromatography can be used for laboratory-scale purification, its utilization on a preparative scale can represent a major cost for the final protein product. Successful separation by affinity chromatography requires that a biospecific ligand is available, and that it is covalently attached to a chromatographic bed material. It is important that the biospecific ligand (antibody, enzyme, or receptor protein) retains its specific binding affinity for the substance of interest (antigen, substrate, or hormone). These interactions typically have high affinities ($K_d < 10_{-6}$ M) yet are reversible when conditions are changed. Due to the specificity of this recognition, it is often possible to obtain 100-, 1.000- or even 100.000-fold increases in purity of a protein sample. The packing material used, called the affinity matrix, must be inert and easily modified. Agarose is the most common substance used as a matrix, in spite of its relative high costs. The ligands, or "affinity tails", that are inserted into the matrix can be genetically engineered to possess a specific affinity. In a process similar to ion exchange chromatography, the desired molecules adsorb to the ligands on the matrix until esorption is carried out *e.g.*, with a high salt concentration, a competition reaction (*e.g.*, imidazole), strong chelating agents and/or low pH. Fouling of the matrix can occur when a large number of impurities are present, therefore, this type of chromatography is usually implemented late in the process. In addition to most common affinity chromatography utilizing HPLC, there are also other techniques which involve affinity, such as affinity precipitation, affinity partitioning of proteins using aqueous two-phase system, foam fractionation and dye ligand chromatography (58).

Affinity Tags

To date, a large number of different fusion partners that range in size from one amino acid to whole proteins capable of selective interaction with ligand immobilized onto a chromatography matrix, have been described. Although a multitude of systems have been introduced, no single affinity fusion partner is ideal for all expression or purification systems. In 1975 scientists introduced a method based on the interaction between the side chains of certain amino acids, especially histidines, on a protein surface and immobilized transition metal ions. Immobilized metal affinity chromatography (IMAC) systems have three basic components: an electron donor group, a solid support and a V metal ion. The metal ion (usually Ni_2^+, CO_2^+, CU_2^+ or Zn_2^+) is restrained in a coordination complex where it still retains significant affinity towards macromolecules. The use of *polyhistidine tags* has been demonstrated in a wide range of host cells including *E. coli, S. cerevisiae,* insect cells as well as in mammalian cells. IMAC is usually performed under non-denaturing conditions, but it is also compatible with non-ionic detergents allowing highly denaturing conditions with urea and guanidium-HC1. Also an organic solvent (isopropanol) can be used to increase the purification efficiency (59). The elution is usually performed by competition with imidazole, lowering pH, or by adding strong chelating agents. IMAC is particularly suitable for preparative group fractionation of complex extracts and biofluids, but can also be used in the high-performance mode. Regardless of the relatively small size of the his-tag, is has been reported recombinant, proteins. *Maltose binding protein* (MBP) from *E. coli* is frequently used as a fusion partner for proteins. MBP (40 kDa) is a periplasmic protein and thereby can be employed to induce the secretion into the periplasm. A mixture of cellulose and starch can be utilized as a ligand and elution can be achieved in the presence of maltose. MBP has reported to increase the solubility of the fusion protein and it has been successfully used vas a C-terminal fusion partner. *Glutathione S-Transferase* (GST)-fusion vectors were first reported by Smith and Jonhson (1988) (60). GSTs are a family of enzymes that can transfer sulfur from glutathione to substances such as nitro and halogenated compounds, leading to their detoxication. GST fusion proteins are bound to immobilized glutathione reduced glutathione. Since GST is a relatively large tag (26 kDa), in many cases it is preferable to remove it by engineering a specific cleavage site. GST can also be utilized under denaturing conditions. However, a possible complication associated with this system is the use of reduced glutathione for elution, since it can affect target proteins containing disulfides (61). *Staphylococcal protein A* is a immunoglobulin-binding receptor on the surface of the gram-positive bacterium *Staphylococcus aureus.* Protein (30 kDa) and its derivative Z shows a specific affinity for the Fc-region of immunoglobulin G. Protein A consists of five repetitive homologous domains (A-E), and each of these domains alone is capable of binding to IgG. The structure of the B domain (from which Z has been derived) has been determined, revealing that the N- and C-, termini of the three-helix bundle structure are solvent exposed, which is supposed to favor an independent folding of the target protein. Analysis of different repeats of Z showed that there is no advantage in using more than two domains. Protein A is secretion competent and fusion proteins can be secreted to the *E. coli* periplasm and in some cases also to the culture medium. Protein A has been reported to be highly soluble and capable of renaturation after being subjected to denaturants such as urea and guanidium HCl. The need for low pH for elution can be circumvented by the use of competitive elution strategies based on engineered competitor proteins. Like protein A, *Staphylococcal protein G,* is a receptor present on the surface of certain strains of *Streptococci.* Protein G is a bifunctional protein having structurally separate regions for affinity to serum albumin and IgG. The serum albumin binding region has three helix-bundle domains, very similar to that of protein A. Elution from a column is usually achieved with low pH or by alternative methods such as high pH, lithium diiodosalisylate and heat (57). Protein G or different parts of the albumin binding domain have been used as affinity tags in protein expressed either intracellularly or as secreted proteins. *Thioredoxin* (Trx, 12 kD), the product of the *E. coli trxA* gene, has been used to increase solubility as well as a fusion partner in *E. coli.* Proteins expressed as thioredoxin fusions are likely to be soluble, since thioredoxin remains soluble even at levels as high as 40 per cent of the total. cellular protein (62). The other obvious benefit associated with the use of thioredoxin is that it provides partial purification *i.e.,* the recombinant protein accumulates in adhesion zones and it can be selectively released by rapid osmotic shock treatment. Thioredoxin also provides an affinity tag for rapid purification, since it specifically bonds to ThioBond™-resin. The resin consists of covalently bound phenylarsine oxide on an agarose-based support to which the thioredoxin's active site diothiol has a high affinity. The Trxsystem has been utilized to produce short amino acid sequences (10-30 aa) which are usually extensively degraded or insoluble when expressed in *E. coil.* Furthermore, a plasmid has been developed for *in vivo* biotinylation of Trx-fusion proteins in *E. coli. FLAG peptide* (about 1 kDa) is an eight amino acid long peptide (63). The sequence of the peptide (Asp- Tyr-Lys-Asp-Asp-Asp-Asp-Lys) is designed for maximum hydrophilicity and contains an enterokinase cleavage site. There are two common monoclonal antibodies raised against this peptide: MI and M2. Antibody M1 binds to the peptide in a calcium-dependent manner, which allows gentle elution by the addition of a chelating agent. For antibody recognition the FLAG peptide must be located on the very N terminal end of the target protein. The M1 antibody recognizes only the four first amino acids of the peptide (Asp-Tyr-Lys-Asp) allowing a shorter tag to be utilized. Antibody M2 is capable of recognizing the FLAG peptide also at other locations in addition to the N-terminal site. Fusion proteins bond by antibody M2 can not be eluted with a chelating agent, but instead by low pH or competition with an excess of FLAG peptide (Brizzard *et al.*, 1994). There are also specific antibodies raised against the FLAG peptide sequence including a methionine at the N-terminus (64). The strong affinity between *biotin* and *avidin* or *streptavidin*. have been used for various detection, immobilization and purification processes. BiotinylatIon of a protein can be achieved by covalent coupling of biotin to its lysine residues. The biotinylation method introduced by Cronan (65) utilize *in vivo* machinery for specific biotinylation which can not be achieved *in vitro*. A 75 residue fragment of transcarboxylase has been shown to be a sufficiently large substrate for biotinylation. Elution can be performed under mild conditions with excess biotin. Denaturing conditions may also be utilized since avidin, as a ligand, is fairly stable allowing purification in the presence of 1 per cent SDS or 8 M urea (65). The Cterminal 101 residues of the *E. coli* biotin carboxyl carrier protein of acetyl-CoA carboxylase, has been utilized as an affinity tag for Fab antibody fragment in *E. coli.* A subunit form of transcaboxylase has also been used as a biotinylated fusion partner in recombinant Semliki Forest virus-infected baby hamster kidney (BHK) and chinese hamster ovarian cells. PinPoint (13 kDa, Promega) binds to streptavidin/avidin or monomeric avidin and can be eluted with biotin. An alternative small affinity tag that binds to streptavidin is Strep (10 aa) which mimics biotin even though it is nonbiotinylated. Strep fusion proteins can be eluted under mild conditions with a biotin analog, named iminobiotin. An improved version of the strep tag is strep-tag II which retains its binding activity also when placed at positions other than the C-terminus. Sometimes it is convenient to have more than one fusion partner. The *Dual affinity fusion* concept, which in addition to providing the possibility for two affinity chromatographic purification steps, can also stabilize the target protein more than is possible with just one fusion partner (57). Rigaut *et al.*, (66) successfully purified several proteins with a tandem affinity purification procedure. The tags used were protein A and calmodulin-binding peptide in combination with a TEV -cleavage site. The first purification step involved protein binding to an IgG matrix, followed by TEV -protease cleavage. The released protein could be separated from the protease by a second affinity chromatography step using calmodulincoated beads. The His6-tag together with the maltose-binding-protein have also been used for double-affinity purification system for several proteins in *E. coli* (67, 68).

Cleavage

In many applications there is no need to remove the tag since it does not interfere with the activity of the protein of interest (69). However, sometimes it is necessary to remove the tag, since it can cause unwanted immuno responses, inactivate the fused target protein or prevent structural determination. Several methods have been described for site-specific cleavage treatment of the fusion partner. Careful upstream design of the fusion protein, construct can facilitate the subsequent purification of the target protein. Furthermore, it may allow for integrated systems involving co-processing of the protein and efficient removal of the affinity fusion partner as well as the protease used for the cleavage. Chemical cleavage methods utilizing, for example, cyanogen bromide and hydroxylamine are relatively inexpensive. Nevertheless, the chemicals are relatively unspecific and the reaction conditions used can cause amino acid side chain modifications, denaturation or partial degradation of the target protein. Enzymatic methods are preferred due to their specificity and milder reaction conditions required. However, the proteases cleaving after a basic residue (enterokinase, thrombin and factor Xa) sometimes display non-specific and unwanted cleavages. IgA-proteinase has been reported to be more specific since it requires a proline in the P2′ position. After cleavage, the target protein can be purified from the tag by affinity chromatography. Protease can also be designed to contain a tag by which it can be separated from the target protein, and thus facilitate the purification (57). For certain applications it is convenient to perform a site-specific cleavage when the fusion protein is still bound on the affinity column. An example of a protein purified by this method is the DNA binding domain of the glucocorticoid receptor fused to protein A. For some applications maintenance of an authentic N-terminus of the protein is required. For this purpose the initiation methionine can be removed by cyanogen bromide or by *in vitro* cleavage *e.g.*, within the sites of specific proteases such as aminopeptidase, enterokinase or factor Xa. The authentic N-terminus can also be obtained by using ubiquitin as a fusion partner.

Analysis of Posttranslational Modifications

Many proteins are subsequently modified in various ways after or during the assembly of the polypeptide chain (70). The terminal methionine can be hydrolyzed, one or more N-terminal residues may be removed and/or polypeptides can be specifically cleaved. Disulfide bonds may be formed by oxidation of two cysteines and certain amino acids, chains can be modified by *e.g.*, hydroxylation, sulfation, acylation, glycosylation and N phosphorylation. Also prosthetic groups, such as lipoate, are covalently attached to some proteins. However, only the analysis techniques concerning three common posttranslational modification *i.e.*, glycosylation, acylation and phosphorylation are reviewed here.

Glycosylation

Many luminal, secreted and membrane proteins, as well as some cytoplasmic proteins, are modified by glycosylation. Together with glycolipids, membrane glycoproteins are responsible for many important functional properties of the eukaryotic cell surface, *e.g.*, cell-cell recognition and adhesion, blood group specific antigens, virus, bacteria and protozoan receptors, transplantation (histo-compatibility) antigens, ion channels and many others (71). In general glycosylation is a complex process and varies in different cell types, and cannot be easily predicted by simple rules. Two types of carbohydrate-protein linkages are found: O-linked and N-linked. O-glycosidic bonds occur between the hydroxyl group of serine or threonine and an amino sugar, whereas N-glycosidic bonds are between the amide nitrogen of asparagine and the C-1 of an amino sugar residue. N-glycosidic glycosylation can occur in the sequence motif of Asn-X-Ser, or Asn-X-Thr, where X can be any amino-acid except proline and asparagine. N-glycans can be subdivided into three distinct groups called 'high mannose type', 'hybrid type', and 'complex type' glucans. The determination of oligosaccharide composition can be demanding since saccharides have very complex structure having branching and anomeric configurations (alpha and beta linkages). The complete characterization of the glycosylation of a glycoprotein entails the determination of three variables: Firstly, the occupancy of potential glycosylation sites; secondly, the type(s) of oligosaccharides present at these sites, and thirdly, the distribution of oligosaccharides structures at each site (72). To study whether the protein is modified by glycosylation, metabolic labelling with radioactive saccharide and/or affinity chromatography (lectin, Con-A) can be utilized. A radioactive sample can be obtained by labeling either metabolically or chemically, or a radioactive sugar nucleotide can be transferred from another saccharide using a glycosyltransferase. In many cases for the analysis of the saccharide composition and structure, it is necessary to release the saccharides from the glycoprotein. Methods used to release saccharides include the enzymatic approach (endo/exoglycosidases), chemical methods and digestion of the protein with proteases. Since the glycoside bond between the hydroxyl group and amino sugar can be disrupted by alkali treatment, O-linked saccharides are released by β-elimination. However, this technique releases other O-linked residues *e.g.*, phosphate. Purified glycopeptides or saccharide moieties can be further analyzed by RP-HPLC, gas-liquid chromatography or thin layer chromatography (TLC). Mono- and disaccharides can also be determinated by paper chromatography. In addition, many inhibitors and comparative substrates can be utilized to alter the glycoconjugates, for example N-linked glycosylation can be prevented by tunicamycin and the elongation of the saccharide chain can be stopped at different stages by other specific inhibitors. Finally, there are many other approaches to analyze oligosaccharides such as the glycolipide anchor method, polysaccharide lyase, the phenolsulfuric acid assay, and mass spectrometry (MS).

Acylation

There are three common types of lipid modifications of cytoplasmic proteins: myristate (C14-saturated fatty acid), palmitate (C16 saturated fatty acid) and isoprenoids (farnesyl, geranyl) (73). Some membrane proteins can also carry a stearate (C18-saturated fatty acid) and glycosylphosphatidylinositol anchor. Modification of the proteins by lipids appears often to be the first membrane binding step. Lipid modifications with myristate or isoprenoids, are attached through chemically stable amine or thioether bonds, respectively, whereas palmitate is attached through a chemically fragile thioester linkage (74). There is no recognition sequence for palmityolation, but often the palmitate is attached to cysteine residues. A conserved eight amino acid sequence is the minimum number of residues that provides an effective signal for myristoylation, but a large number of eukaryotic proteins are myristoylated at their N-terminal glycine-residue *via* amide linkage. Prenyl groups are attached to C-terminal cysteine residues *via* a thioester linkage. Preliminary indications that a protein is acylated can be provided by the incorporation of radiolabeled fatty acids or by mass spectrometry (MS). Acylation of a protein can be indicated when discrepancies between the observed molecular weight of a peptide and the calculated mass of the amino acids corresponds to the mass of an acyl sequence. The specific modified amino acid residues can be identified by tandem mass spectrometry (MS/MS) of proteolytic peptides. The incorporated fatty acid can also be identified by gas chromatography after hydrolysis and methyl esterification (74). A sequential hydrolysis with acid, KOH/ methanol and hydroxylamine might give information about the nature of the bonds between the acyl-group and the protein. Furthermore, the released fatty acids can then be identified by liquid chromatography or TLC. Nuclear magnetic resonance (NMR) has been used to study C-terminal alkylation with isoprenoid farnesyl or geranylgeranyl groups (75).

Phosphorylation

Phosphorylation is generally considered to be the most prevalent posttranslational modification of proteins. It has been shown that many cellular processes such as signal transduction, enzymatic activities, protein translation and cell division are regulated by phosphorylation and dephosphorylation (76). Proteins can be phosphorylated at serine, threonine and tyrosine to form Ophosphomonoesters.Besides the commonly occurring phosphorylated amino acid residues in proteins, phosphomono- and phosphodiesters have been found to be attached to sugar residues of some oligosaccharide side chains. One of the best known examples of the functional phosphate esters is the targeting of some hydrolytic enzymes to lysosome by mannose residues that are phosphorylated at the C-6 hydroxyl group, known as the mannose 6-P recognition signal. With radioactive labelling it is possible to determine if the protein is modified by phosphorylation. Other techniques to detect possible phosphorylation are dephosphorylation with phosphatases and immunodetection with antiphosphoserine/threonine/tyrosine antibodies. To further study the function of phosphorylation it is necessary to identify the exact phosphorylation sites. This can be approached by site-directed mutagenesis, tryptic phosphopeptide mapping, followed by Edman degradation or from pure peptide samples by mass spectrometry. To analyze the type(s) of amino acids phosphorylated, the protein is subjected to acid hydrolysis, and phosphorylated amino acids are separated by chromatographic and/or electrophoretic systems. In addition to peptide bonds phosphodiester bonds are also unstable under the reaction conditions that lead to the release of free ($_{32}$P) phosphate. As a consequence, hydrolysis times are critical as usually no more than 20 per cent of the radioactivity can be recovered as free phosphoamino acids. Sometimes one-dimensional migration is sufficient to separate all three phosphoamino acids (77) but often two-dimensional (2D) analysis is required. 2D-systems can consist of two successive chromatography (78), two successive electrophoresis or an electrophoresis followed by chromatography. Peptide mapping or peptide fingerprinting is a powerful technique to analyze phosphoamino acid composition as well as other post translational modifications (*i.e.*, glycosylation, fatty acid acylation, methylation and acetylation). Phosphopeptide mapping (PPM) of a digested protein can give an overall view of how many sites are phosphorylated or it can be used to study the effects of different treatments and the site-directed mutagenesis on the relation of phosphorylated peptides. 2D-mapping is an extremely sensitive technique that requires only minor amounts of metabolically labeled product. Resolving the peptide mixture in two dimensions often yields subtle but important clues about peptide composition. Because cellulose is an inert material, the peptides can be recovered from the plate for further analysis, such as amino acid analysis or Edman degradation. Two-dimensional electrophoresis is an effective method for the analysis of abroad range of complex protein samples, and post translational modifications like phosphorylation. The technique sorts proteins into two dimensions according to their isoelectric points (IEF) and sizes (SDS-PAGE). Drawbacks of this method are its extreme sensitivity to salts and other impurities as well as its unsuitability for membrane proteins. An improved variation of 2D electrophoresis utilizes immobilized pH gradients by which the inconsistencies among carrier ampholytes are circumvented (79).

Mass Spectrometry (MS) is a rapid and extremely sensitive tool for the determination of post translational modifications, including phosphorylation (80). By utilizing techniques such as matrix-assisted laser descrption/ionization (MALDI) and electrospray ionization (ESI) MS is able to analyze a sample below the picomolar level. MS with collision-induced dissociation (CID) after phosphopeptide precursor-ion scan of m/z of 79 can be utilized to sequence phosphopeptides (81). However, identification can sometimes be ambiguous, especially when a protein/peptide exists in complex mixtures. Peptide characteristics can make the identification process difficult or occasionally impossible, *i.e.*, negatively charged peptides may be poorly ionized in the positive mode thus preventing sequence analysis by CID MS. Moreover, large peptides will not release an informative fragmentation pattern and small peptides (under 600 kDa) are more likely to be lost within the region of matrix signals. To avoid adventitious formation of acrylamide, adducts during electrophoresis: alkylation with iodo-acetamide, 4-vinylpyridine and acrylamide can be performed prior to SDS-P AGE. The peptides for MS can be purified by RPHPLC either off- or on-line. Phosphopeptides can be also purified by binding them to an ironchelating column (IMAC). MS can be used to identify phosphorylation sites alone or in combination with other methods such as hosphopeptide mapping, 2D- electrophoresis and Edman degradation. Phosphoprotein or hosphopeptides prepared by enzymatic (phosphatase treatment) or chemical degradation (β-elimination) can be identified by their m/z of 79 (PO_3)- or 97 (H_2PO_4)- mass difference compared to the peptides expected from the sequence (82). An elegant way of determining phosphorylation sites utilizes on-line electrospray mass spectrometry, connected to an IMAC column and/or micro liquid chromatography column.

References

1. Sassenfeld, H.M. (1990). Engineering proteins for purification. *Trends Biotechnol.*, 8: 88-93.

2. Nilsson, B., Forsberg, G., Moks, T., Hartmanis, M. and Uhlen, M. (1992). Fusion proteins in biotechnology and structural biology. *Curr. Opin. Struct. Biol.*, 2: 569-575.

3. Hodgson, J. (1993). Expression systems: A user's guide. *Biotechnology*, 11: 887-893.

4. Baneyx, F. (1999). Recombinant protein expression in *Escherichia coli*. *Curr. Opin. Biotechnol.*, 10: 411-421.

5. LaVallie, E.R. and McCoy, J.M. (1995). Gene fusion expression system in *Escherichia coli*. *Curr. Opin. Biotechnol.*, 6: 501-506.

6. Lilie, H., Schwarz, E. and Rudolph, R. (1998). Advances in refolding of proteins produced in *E. coli*. *Curr. Opin. Biotechnol.*, 9: 497-501.

7. De Bernardez Clark, E. (1998). Refolding of recombinant proteins. *Curr. Opin. Biotechnol.*, 9: 157-163.

8. Murby, M., Uhlén, M. and Stãhl, S. (1996). Upstream strategies to minimize proteolytic degratation upon recombinant production in *Escherichia coli*. *Protein Expr. Purif.*, 7: 129-136.

9. Patra, A.K., Mukhopadhyay, R., Mukhija, R., Krishnan, A., Garg, L.C. and Panda, A.K. (2000). Optimization of inclusion body solubinization and renaturation of recombinant human growth hormone from *Escherichia coil*. *Protein Expr. Purif.*, 18: 182-192.

10. Peränen, J., Rikkonen, M., Hyvönen, M. and Kääräinen, L. (1996). T7 vectors with a modified T7*lac* promoter for expression of proteins in *Escherichia coli*. *Anal. Biochem.*, 236: 371-373.

11. Valax, P. and Georgiou, G. (1993). Molecular characterization of beta-lactamase, inclusion bodies produced in *Escherichia coli*. 1. Composition. *Biotechnol. Progr.*, 9: 539-547.

12. Wilkinson, D.L. and Harrison, R.G. (1991). Predicting the solubility of recombinant proteins in *Escherichia coli*. *Biotechnology*, 9: 443-448.

13. Georgiou, G. and Valax, P. (1999). Isolating inclusion bodies from bacteria. *Methods. Enzymol.*, 306: 48-58.

14. Zhang, Y., Olsen, D.R., Nguyen, K.B., Olsen, P.S., Rhodes, E.T. and Mascarenhas, D. I. (1998). Expression of eukaryotic proteins in soluble form in *Escherichia coli*. *Protein Expr. Purif.*, 12: 159-165.

15. Samuelsson, E., Moks, T., Nilsson, B. and Uhlén, M. (1994). Enhanced *in vitro* refolding of insulin-like growth factor using a solubilizing fusion partner. *Biochemistry*, 33: 4207-4211.

16. Wall, J.G. and Plückthun, A. (1995). Effects of overexpressing folding modulators on the *in vivo* folding of heterologous proteins in *Escherichia coli*. *Curr. Opin. Biotechnol.*, 6: 507-516.

17. Frangioni, J.V. and Neel, B.G. (1992). Solubilization and purification of enzymatically active glutathione s-transferase (pGEX) fusion proteins. *Anal. Biochem.* 210: 179-187.

18. Weiss, E., Chatellier, J. and Orfanoudakis, G. (1994). *In vivo* biotinylated recombinant antibodies: Construction, characterization, and application of abifunctional Fab-BCCP fusion proteins produced in *Escherichia coli. Protein Expr. Purif.*, 5: 509-517.

19. Goffeau, A., Aert, R., Agostini-Carbone, M.L., Ahmed, A., Aigle, M., Alberghina, L., Albermann, K., Albers, M., Aldea, M., Alexandraki, D., Aljinovic, G., Allen, E., Altmann, R., Alt-Mörbe, J., André, B., Andrews, S., Ansorge, W., Antoine, G., Anwar, R., Aparicio A. *et al.* (1997). *Saccharomyces cerevisiae* Genome. *Nature* 387 (6632 Suppl.): 1-105.

20. Goodly, A.R. (1993). The production of heterologous plasma proteins. *Trends Biotechnol.*, 11: 430-433.

21. Fleer, R. (1992). Engineering yeast for high level expression. *Curr. Opin. Biotechnol.*, 3: 486-496.

22. Suntio, T., Shmelev, A., Lund, M. and Makarow, M. (1999). The sorting determinant guiding Hsp150 to the COPI-independent transport pathway in yeast. *J. Cell Sci.*, 112: 3889-3898.

23. Chung, B.H., Seo, D.J. and Nam, S.W. (1999). High-Ievel secretory production of recombinant human lipocortin-1 by *Saccharomyces cerevisiae. Proc. Biochem.*, 35: 97-101.

24. Cartwright, C.P., Zhu, Y.S. and Tipper, D.J. (1992). Efficient secretion in yeast based on fragments from K1 killer preprotoxin. *Yeast*, 8: 261-272.

25. Orci, L., Stamnes, M., Ravazzola, M., Amherdt, M., Perrelet, A., Söllner, T.H. and Rothman, J.E. (1997). Bidirectional transport bydistinct populations of COPI-coated vesicles. *Cell*, 90: 335-349.

26. Conibear, E. and Stevens, T.H. (2000). Vps52p, Vps53p and Vps54p from a novel multi subunit complex required for protein sorting at the yeast late Golgi. *Mol. Biol. Cell*, 11: 305-323.

27. Walter, P. and Johnson, A.E. (1994). Signal sequence recognition and protein targeting to the endoplasmic reticulum membrane. *Annu. Rev. Cel. Biol.*, 10: 87-119.

28. Matlack, K.E.S., Misselwitz, B., Plath, K. and Rapoport, T.A. (1999). BiP acts as a molecular ratchet during posttranslational transport of prepro factor across the ER membrane. *Cell*, 97: 553- 565.

29. Varki, A. (1998). Factors controlling the glyco-sylation potential of the Golgi apparatus. *Trends Cell. Biol.*, 8: 34-40.

30. Lee, J., Choi, S.I., Jang, J.S., Jang, K., Moon, J. W., Bae, C.S., Yang, D.S. and Seong, B.L. (1999). Novel secretion system of recombinant *Saccharomyces cerevisiae* using an N-terminus residue of human IL-IB as secretion enhancer. *Biotechnol. Prog.*, 15: 884-890.

31. Shusta, E.V., Bockhaus, J.A., Voegler, A.C. and Wittrup, K.D. (1998). Increasing the secretory capacity of *Saccharomyces cerevisiae* for production of single-chain antibody fragments. *Nat. Biotechnol.*, 16: 773-777.

32. Jarvis, D.L., Weinkauf, C. and Guarino, L.A. (1996). Immediate-early baculovirus vectors for foreign gene expression in transformed or infected insect cells. *Protein Expr. Purif.*, 8: 191-203.

33. Farrell, P.J., Lu, M., Prevost, J., Brown, C., Behie, L. and Iatrou, K. (1998). High-level expression of secreted glycoproteins in transformed lepidopteran insect cells using a novel expression vector. *Biotechnol. Bioeng.*, 60: 656-663.

34. Summers, M.D. and Smith, G.E. (1988). A manual of methods for baculovirus vectors and insect cell culture procedures. *Texas Agricultural Experiment Station, bulletin* No. 1555, College Station, Texas, 57 pages.

35. Naggie, S. and Bentley, W.E. (1998). Appearance of protease activities coincides with p10 and polyhedrin-driven protein production in the baculovirus expression system: Effects on yield. *Biotechnol. Prog.*, 14: 227-232.

36. Bonning, B.C., Roelvink, P.W., Vlak, J.M., Possee, R.D. and Hammock, B.D. (1994). Superior expression of juvenile hormone esterase and β-galactosidase from the basic protein promoter of *Autographa californica* nuclear polyhedrosis virus compared to the p 10 protein and polyherdin promoters. *J. Gen. Virol.*, 75: 1551-1556.

37. Kitts, P. and Possee, R. (1993). A method for producing recombinant baculovirus expression vectors at high frequency. *BioTechniques*, 14: 810- 817.

38. Leusch, M.S., Lee, S.C. and Olins, P.O. (1995). A novel host-vector system for direct selection of recombinant baculoviruses (bacmids) in *Escherichia coli. Gene*, 160: 191-194.

39. Klaassen, C.H.W., Bovee-Geurts, P.H.M., DeCaluwe, G.L.J. and DeGrip, W.J. (1999). Large-scale production and purification of functional recombinant bovine rhdopsin with the use of the baculovirus expression system. *Biochem. J.*, 342: 293-300.

40. Bonning, B.C., Roelvink, P.W., Vlak, J.M., Possee, R.D. and Hammock, B.D. (1994). Superior expression of juvenile hormone esterase and β-galactosidase from the basic protein promoter of *Autographa californica* nuclear polyhedrosis virus compared to the p10 protein and polyherdin promoters. *J. Gen. Virol.*, 75: 1551-1556.

41. Geisse, S. and Kocher, H.P. (1999). Protein expression in mammalian and insect cell systems. *Methods Enzymol.*, 306: 19-41.

42. Wyatt, L., Moss, B. and Rozenblatt, S. (1995). Replication deficient vaccinia virus encoding bacteriophage T7 RNA polymerase for transient gene expression in mammalian cells. *Virology*, 210: 202-205.

43. Himly, M., Pfleiderer, M., Holzer, G., Fischer,U., Hannak, E., Falkner, F.G. and Dorner, F. (1998). Defective vaccinia virus as a biologically safe tool for the erproduction of recombinant human secretory proteins. *Protein Expr. Purif.*, 14: 317-326.

44. Smerdou, C. and Liljestrom, P. (1999). Two-helper RNA system for production of recombinant Semliki Forst virus particles. *J. Virol.*, 73: 1092-1098.

45. Dryga, S.A, Dryga, O.A. and Schlesinger, S. (1997). Identification of mutation in a Sindbis virus variant to estabilish persistant infection in BHK cell: The importance of a mutation in the nsP2 gene. *Virology*, 228:74-83.

46. Ohno, K., Sawai, K., Iiijima, Y., Levin, B. and Meruelo, D. (1997). Cell-specific targeting of Sindbis virus vectors displaying IgG binding domains of proteins A. *Nat. Biotechnol.*, 15:763-767.

47. Cichna, M., Markl, P. and Huber, J.F. (1995). Determination of true octanol-water partition coefficients by means of solvent generated liquid-liquid chromatography. *J. Pharm. Biomed. Anal.*, 13: 339-351.

48. Zeng, X. and Ruckenstein, E. (1999). Membrane chromatography: preparation and application to protein separation. *Biotechnol. Prog.*, 15: 1003-1019.

49. Choudhary, G. and Horváth, C. (1996). Ion-exchange chromatography. *Methods Enzymol.*, 270: 47-82.

50. Stålberg, J. (1999). Retention models for ions in chromatography. *J. Chromatogr. A.*, 855: 3-55.

51. Zhou, D.P. Malissard, M., Berger, *E.G.* and Rennet, T. (2000). Secretion and purification of recombinant beta 1-4 galactotransferase from insect cells using pFme-protA, a novel transposition based baculovirus transfer vector. *Arc. Biochem. Biophys.*, 374: 3-7.

52. Nimura, N., Itoh, R., Kinoshita, T., Nagae, N. and Nomura, M. (1992). Fast protein separation by reversed-phase high performance liquid chromatography on octadecylsilyl-bonded non-porous silica gel. *J. Chromatogr.*, 585: 207-211.

53. Van Dijk, J.A.P.P. and Smit, J.A.M. (2000). Size-exclusion chromatograhpy-multiangle laser light scattering analysis of β-lactoglobulin and bovine serum albumin in aqueous solution with added salt. *J. Chromatogr.*, 867: 105-112.

54. Pujar, N.S. and Zydney, A.L. (1998). Electrostatic effects on protein partitioning in size-exclusion chromatography and membrane ultra-filtration. *J. Chromatogr.*, 796: 229-238.

55. Müller, C. and Rinas, U. (1999). Renaturation of heterodimeric platelet-derived growth factor from inclusion bodies of recombinant *Escherichia coli* using size-exclusion chromatography. *J. Chromatogr.*, 855: 203-213.

56. Batas, B. and Chaudhuri, J.B. (1999). Considerations of sample application and elution during size-exclusion chromatography-based protein refolding. *J. Chromatogr.* 864: 229-236.

57. Nilsson, B., Ståhl, S., Lundeberg, J., Uhlén, M. and Nygren, P. Å. (1997). Affinity fusion strategies for detection, purification, and

immobilization of recombinant proteins. *Protein Expr. Purif.*, 11: 1-16.

58. Roshino, K., Taniguchi, M., Kitao, T., Morohashi, S. and Sasakura, T. (1998). Preparation of a new thermo-responsive adsorbent with maltose as a ligand and its application to affinity precipitation. *Biotechnol. Bioeng.*, 60: 568-579.

59. Franken, K.L.M.C., Hiemstra, R.S., van Meijgaarden, K.E., Subronto, Y., den Hartigh, J., Ottenhoff, T.R.M. and Drijfhout, J.W. (2000). Purification of Ris-tagged proteins by immobilized chelated affinity chromatography: the benefits from the use of organic solvent. *Protein Expr. Purif.*, 18: 95-99.

60. Smith, D.B. and Jonhson, K.S. (1988). Single-step purification of polypeptides expressed in *Escherichia coli* as fusion with glutathione S-transferase. *Gene*, 67: 31-40.

61. Sassenfeld, H.M. (1990). Engineering proteins for purification. *Trends Biotechnol.*, 8: 88-93.

62. Yasukawa, T., Kanei-Ishii, C., Maekawa, T., Fujimoto, J., Yamamoto, T. and Ishii, S. (1995). Increase of solubility of foreign proteins in *Escherichia coli* by coproduction of the bacterial thioredoxin. *J. Biol. Chem.*, 270: 25328-25331.

63. Hopp, T.R., Prickett, K.S., Price, V.L., Libby, R.T., March, C.J., Cerretti, D.P., Urdal, D.L. and Conlon, P.J. (1988). A short polypeptide marker sequence useful for recombinant protein identification and purification. *Biotechnology*, 6: 1204-1210.

64. Chubet, R.G. and Brizzard, B.L. (1996). Vectors for expression and secretion of FLAG epitope-tagged proteins in mammalian cells. *Biotechniques*, 20: 136-141.

65. Cronan, J.E. (1990). Biotination of proteins *in vivo:* A post-translational modification to label, purify, and study proteins. *J. Biol. Chem.*, 265: 10327-10333.

66. Rigaut, G., Shevchenko, A., Rutz, B., Wilm, M., Mann, M. and Seraphin, B. (1999). A generic protein purification method for protein complex characterization and proteome exploration. *Nat. Biotechnol.*, 17: 1030-1032.

67. Pryor, K.D. and Leiting, B. (1997). High-level expression of soluble protein in *Escherichia coli* using a His6-tag and maltose-

binding-protein double-affinity fusion system. *Protein Expr. Purif.*, 10: 309-319.

68. Stempfer, G., Höll-Neugebauer, B. and Rudolph, R. (1996). Improved refolding of an immobilized fusion protein. *Nat. Biotechnol.*, 14: 329-334.

69. Wold, F. (1981). *In vivo* chemical modification of proteins (post-translational modification). *Ann.Rev. Biochem.*, 50: 783-814.

70. Parekh, R.B. (1991). Effects of glycosylation on protein function. *Curr. Opin. Struct. Biol.*, 1: 750-754.

71. Ashford, D.A. (1992). Carbohydrate analysis. *Curr. Opin. Biotechnol.*, 3: 45-48.

72. Solski, P.A., Quilliam, A., Coats, S.G., Der, C.J. and Buss, J.J.E. (1996). Targeting proteins to membranes using signal sequence for lipid modification. *Methods Enzymol.*, 250: 435-454.

73. Bizzozero, O.A. (1995). Chemical analysis of acylation sites and species. *Methods Enzymol.*, 250: 361-379.

74. Anderegg, R.J., Betz, R., Carr, S.A., Crabb, J.W. and Duntze, W. (1988). Structure of *Saccharomyces cerevisiae* mating hormone factor. Identification of S-famesyl cysteine as a structural component. *J. Biol. Chem.*, 263: 18236-18240.

75. Hunter, T. (1995). Protein kinase and phos-phatases: The Yin and Yang of protein phospho-rylation and signaling. *Cell*, 80: 225-236.

76. Jelinek, T. and Weber, M.J. (1993). Optimization of the resolution of phosphoamino acids by one-dimensional thin-layer electrophoresis. *Biotechniques*, 15: 628-630.

77. Grimm, S.L. and Nordeen, S.K. (1999). Altemative procedure for two-dimensional separation of phosphoamino acids. *Biotechniques*, 27: 62-64.

78. Görg, A., Postel, W. and Günther, S. (1988). The current state of two-dimensional electrophoresis with immobilized pH gradients. *Electrophoresis*, 9: 531-546.

79. Costello, C.E. (1999). Bioanalytic applications of mass spectrometry. *Curr. Opin. Biotechnol.*, 10: 22-28.

80. Carr, S.A., Huddleston, M.J. and Annan, R.S. (1996). Selective detection and sequencing of phosphopeptides at the femtomole level by mass spectrometry. *Anal. j Biochem.*, 239: 180-192.

81. Neubauer, G. and Mann, M. (1999). Mapping of phosphorylation sites of gel-isolated proteins by nanoelectrospray tandem mass spectrometry: Potentials and limitations. *Anal. Chem.*, 71: 235-242.

Appendices

Available Biotechnology Drugs

Appendix 1: Approved Biotechnology Drugs 2002

Product	*Company*	*Application (Use)*	*Approval Date*
Abbott HTLV- I/ HTLV-II EIA	Abbott Laboratories	EIA for detection of HTLV-I/HTLV-II antibodies in serum or plasma	Aug 1997
Abelcet® (amphotericin B lipid complex injection)	The Liposome Company	Treatment of invasive fungal infections in patients who are refractory to or intolerant of conventional amphotericin B (lipid-complex drug delivery system)	Nov 1995
Actimmune® (Interferon gamma -1b)	Connectics Corporation	Treatment of chronic granulomatous disease	Dec 1990
Activase® (Alterplase recombinant)	Genentech	Treatment of acute myocardial infarction	Nov 1987
		Acute massive pulmonary embolism	June 1990
		Acute ischemic stroke wihtin first three hours of symptom onset	June 1996

Contd...

Appendix 1–Contd...

Product	*Company*	*Application (Use)*	*Approval Date*
Adagen® (adenosine deaminase)	Enzon	Treatment of severe combined immunodeficiency disease (SCID)	March 1990
Albutein® (human albumin)	Alpha Therapeutic Corp.	Treatment of hypovolmeic shock; an adjunct in hemodialysis; in cardiopulmonary bypass procedures	Jan 1986
Alferon N® (interferon alfa-N3, humaan leukocyte derived)	Interferon Sciences	Treatment of genital warts	Oct 1989
Alphanate® (human antihemophilic factor)	Alpha Therapeutic Corp.	Treatment of hemophilia A or acquired Factor VII deficiency	Feb 1997
AlphaNine® SD (virus-filtered human coagulation Factor IX)	Alpha Therapeutic Corp.	Prevention and control of bleeding in patients with Factor IX deficiency due to hemophilia B	July 1996
AmBisome® (lipo-somal amphoteri B)	NeXstar Pharmaceuticals	Primary treatment for presumed fungal infections in patients with depressed immune function and fevers of unknown origin (FUO)	Aug 1997
AMPHOTEC® (lipid-based colloidal dispersion of amphotericin B)	SEQUUS Pharmaceuticals	Second-line treatment of invasive aspergillosis infections	Nov 1996
Apligraf® (graftskin)	Organogenesis	Treatment of venous leg ulcers	May 1998

Contd...

Appendix 1–Contd...

Product	*Company*	*Application (Use)*	*Approval Date*
Avonex® (recombinant interferon beta 1-alpha)	Biogen	Treatment of relapsing forms of multiple sclerosis	May 1996
BeneFix™ Coagulation Factor IX (recombinant)	Genetics Institute	Treatment of hemophilia B	Feb 1997
Betaseron® (recombinant interferon beta 1-B)	Berlex Laboratories / Chiron	Treatment of relapsing, remitting multiple sclerosis	Aug 1993
Bioclate™ (recombinant antihemophilic factor)	Centeon	Treatment of hemophilia A for the prevention and control of hemorrhagic episodes; perioperative management of patients with hemophilia A	Dec 1993
BioTropin™	Biotech General	Treatment of human growth hormone deficiency in children	May 1995
Carticel™ (autologous cultured chondrocytes)	Genzyme	Reconstruction of knee cartilage damage	Aug 1997
Ceredase®/Cerezyme® (alglucerase/recombinant alglucerase)	Gnezyme	Treatment of type I Gaucher's disease	April 1991 May 1994
Chiron RIBA® HCV 3.0 Strip Immunoblot Assay	Chiron/Johnson & Johnson	Detection of antibodies to hepatitis C in human serum or plasma	Feb 1999

Contd...

Appendix 1–Contd...

Product	Company	Application (Use)	Approval Date
CytoGam® (CMV immune globulin IV)	MedImmune Inc.	Prevention of cytomegalovirus (CMV) in kidney transplant patients; prevention of CMV disease associated with kidney, lung, liver, pancreas and heart transplants	April 1990 Dec 1998
DaunoXome® (liposomal form of the chemotherapeutic agent daunorubicin)	NeXstar Pharmaceuticals	Firt-line treatment for HIV-related Kaposi's sarcoma	April 1996
Depocyt™	Depotech (Skye Pharma)/Chiron	Treatment of lymphomatous meningitis	April 1999
Doxil® (liposomal formulation of doxorubicin hydrochloride)	Alza	Second-line therapy for Kaposi's sarcoma in AIDS paritents; metastatic carcinoma of the ovary in patients with disease that is refractory to both paclitaxel- and platinum-based chemotherpy regiments	Nov 1995 June 1999
Enbrel® (etanercept)	Immunex	Reduction in signs and symptoms of moderately to severly active rheumatoid arthiritis in patients who have had an inadequate response to one or more disease-modifying antirheumatic drugs; treatment of polyarticular course juvenile rheumatoid arthritis	Nov 1998 May 1999
Engerix-B® (recombinant Hepatitis B vaccine)	SmithKline Beecham	Hepatitis B vaccine; adults with chronic hepatitis C infection	Sep 1989 Aug 1998

Contd...

Appendix 1–Contd...

Product	*Company*	*Application (Use)*	*Approval Date*
Epogen® (epoetin alfa)	Amgen	Treatment of anemia associated with chronic renal failure and anemia in Retrovir-treated HIV-infected patients; pediateric use	June 1989 July 1999
Fertinex™	Serono Laboratories	Treatment of female infertility to stimulate ovulation in women with ovulatory disorders and in women undergoing assisted reproductive technologies	Aug 1996
Follistim™ (follitropin beta for injection)	Organon	Recombinant follicle-stimulating hormone for treatment of infertility	Sep 1997
Geret®	Serono Laboratories	Treatment of growth hormone deficiency in children with growth failure	Oct 1997
GenoTropin®	Phermacia & Upjohn	Treatment of growth hormone deficiency in children; growth hormone deficiency in adults	Aug 1995 Nov 1997
Gonal-F® (follitropin alfa)	Serono Laboratories	Treatment of functional infertility not due to primary ovarian failure	Sep 1998
Helixate® (recombinant antihemophilic factor)	Centeon	Treatment of hemophilia in which there is a demonstrated deficiency of activity of the plasma clotting factor, Factor VIII; also for treatment of hemophilia A in certain patients with inhibitors to Factor VIII	Feb 1994

Contd...

Appendix 1–Contd...

Product	Company	Application (Use)	Approval Date
Herceptin® (trastuzumab)	Genetech	Treatment of patients with metastatic breast cancer whose tumors over express the HER2 protein	Sep 1998
Hextend® (hetastarch)	BioTime	Plasma volume expander for treatment of hypovolemia during surgery	March 1999
Humalog® (recombinant insulin)	Eli Lilly	Treatment of diabetes	June 1996
Humate-P® (antihemophilic factor/von Willerbrand factor complex-human)	Centeon	Treatment and prevention of bleeding episodes in hemophilia A adult patients; spontaneous and trauma-induced bleeding episodes in severe von Willebrand disease in adult and pediatric patients, and in mild and moderate von Willebrand disease where use of desmopressin is known or suspected to be inadequate	Apr-99
Humatrope®	Eli Lilly	Treatment of growth hormone deficiency in children; somatotropin deficiency syndrome in adults	March 1997 August 1996
Humulin® recombinant human insulin)	Eli Lilly	Treatment of diabetes	Oct 1982

Contd...

Appendix 1–Contd...

Product	Company	Application (Use)	Approval Date
Infergen® (interferon alfacon-1)	Amgen	Treatment of hepatitis C (HCV) in patients 18 years or older with compensated liver disease who have anti-HCV serum antibodies and/or the presence of HCV RNA; subsequent treatment of HCV-infected patients who have tolerated an initial course of interferon therapy	Oct 1997 Dec 1999
Integrelin™ (eptifibatide for injection)	CORTherapeutics/ Schering-Plough	Treatment of patients with acute coronary syndrome and angioplasty; including patients who are to be managed medically and those undergoing percutaneous coronary intervention	May 1998 Sept 1999
Intron A® (alpha-interferon)	Schering-Plough	Treatment of hairy cell leukemia; genital warts; AIDS- related Kaposi's sarcoma; non-A, non-B hepatitis; hepatitis B; chronic malignant melanoma; extended therapy for chronic viral hepatitis C; treatment for follicular lymphoma in conjunction with chemotherapy; treatment of hepatitis B in pediatric patients	June 1986 June 1988 Nov 1988 Feb 1991 July 1992 Dec 1995 March 1997 Nov 1997 Aug 1998
Kogenate® (recombinant antihemophilic factor)	Bayer	Replaces blood-clotting Factor VIII for the treatment of hemophilia A	Sept 1989

Contd...

Appendix 1–Contd...

Product	*Company*	*Application (Use)*	*Approval Date*
Leukine® (yeast-derived GM-CSF)/Leukine Liquid	Immunex	Treatment of autologous bone marrow transplantation; treatment of white blood cell toxicities following induction chemotherapy in older patients with acute myelogenous leukemia; for use following allogenic bone marrow transplantation from HLA-matched related donors; for use mobilizing peripheral blood progenitor cells and for use after PBPC 1 transplantation; (Leukine Liquid) ready to use formulation multidose vial	March 1991 Sept 1995 Nov 1995 Dec 1995 Nov 1996
Luestatin™ (cladribine or 2-CDA)	Ortho Biotech	First-line treatment of hairy cell leukemia	March 1993
Luxiq™	Connetics	Relief of inflammatory and pruritic manifestation of corticosteroid responsive dermatoses of the scalp	Feb 1999
LYMErix™ (recombinant OspaA)	SmithKline Beecham Biologicals	Prevention of Lyme disease	Dec 1998
Nabi-HB™ (hepatitis B immune globulin-human)	Nabi	Treatment of acute exposure to HbsAg, perinatal exposure of infants born to HbsAg-positive mothers, sexual exposure to HbsAg-positive persons and household exposure of infants to persons with acute hepatitis B	Mar-99

Contd...

Appendix 1–Contd...

Product	Company	Application (Use)	Approval Date
Neupogen® (Filgrastim)	Amgen	Treatment of chemotherapy-induced neutropenia; bone marrow transplant accompanied neutropenia; severe chronic neutropenia; autologous bone marrow transplant engraftment or failure; mobilization of autologous PBPCs post chemotherapy	Feb 1991 June 1994 Dec 1994 Dec 1995 April 1998
Neumega® (Oprelvekm)	Genetics Institute	Prevention of severe chemotherapy-induced thrombocytopenia in cancer patients	Nov 1997
Norditropin®	Novo Nordisk	Treatment of growth hormone deficiency in children	May 1995
Novolin® (recombinant human insulin)	Novo Nordisk	Treatment of diabetes	Oct 1982
NovoSeven® (coagulation factor VIIa)	Novo Nordisk	Treatment of bleeding episodes in hemophilia A or B patients with inhibitors to Factor VIII or Factor IX	Mar-99
Nutropin®/Nutropin AQ® (somatropin rDNA)	Genentech	Treatment of growth hormone deficiency in children; growth hormone deficiency in adults; growth failure associated with chronic renal insufficiency prior to kidney transplantation; short stature associated with Turner Syndrome, to improve spine bone mineral density observed in childhood onset adult growth hormone deficient patients and to increase serum alkaline phosphatase	Nov 1993 Jan 1994 Jan 1996 Dec 1996 Dec 1999

Contd...

Appendix 1–Contd...

Product	*Company*	*Application (Use)*	*Approval Date*
Nutropin Depot™ (somatropin for injectable suspension)	Genentech/ Alkermes	Long-acting dosage form of recombinant growth hormone (one or two doses month) for pediatric growth hormone deficiency	Dec 1999
Oncaspar® PEG-L-asparaginase)	Enzon/Rhone-Poulene Rorer	Treatment of acute lymphoblastic leukemia in patients who are hypersensitive to native forms of L-asparaginase	Feb 1994
Ontak® (denileukin diftitox)	Ligand Pharmaceuticals	Treatment of patients with persistent or recurrent cutaneous T-cell lymphoma whose malignant cells express the CD25 component of the interleukin-2 receptor	Feb 1999
Orthoclone OKT3® (Muromonab-CD3)	Ortho Biotech	Reversal of acute kidney transplant rejection	June 1986
Panretin® (alitretinoin)	Ligand Pharmaceuticals	The topical treatment of cutaneous lesions of patients with AIDS-related Kaposi's sarcoma	Feb 1999
Photofrin® Porfimer sodium)	Ligand Pharmaceuticals (licensed from QLT Phototherа-peutics)	Palliative treatment of totally and partially obstructing cancers of esophagus	Nov 1995
Pradin™ (repaglinide)	Novo Nordisk	Anti-diabetic agent for treatment of Type 2 diabetes	Dec 1997

Contd...

Appendix 1–Contd...

Product	*Company*	*Application (Use)*	*Approval Date*
Procrti®	Ortho Biotech	Treatment of anemia in AZT-treated HIV-infected patients; anemia in cancer patients on chemotherapy; for use in anemic patients scheduled to undergo elective noncardiac nonvascular surgery	Dec 1990 April 1993 Dec 1996
Proleukin, IL-2® (Aldesleukin)	Chiron	Treatment of kidney carcinoma/treatment of metastatic melanoma	May 1992 Jan 1998
Protropin® (somatrem)	Genentech	Treatment of growth hormone deficiency in children	Oct 1985
PROVIGIL® (modafinil) Tablets	Cephalon	To improve wakefulness in patients with excessive daytime sleepiness (EDS) associated with narcolepsy	Dec 1998
Pulmozyme® (dornase, alfa recombinant)	Genentech	Treatment of mild to moderate cystic fibrosis; advanced cystic fibrosis; pediatric use in infants 3 months to 2 years and children 2 to 4 years old	Dec 1993 Dec 1996 March 1998
Rebetron™	Schering-Plough	Combination therapy for treatment of chronic hepatitis C in patients with compensated liver disease who have relapsed following alpha-interferon treatment; treatment of chronic hepatitis C in patients with compensated liver disease previously untreated with alpha interferon therapy	June 1998 Dec 1998

Contd...

Appendix 1–Contd...

Product	*Company*	*Application (Use)*	*Approval Date*
Recombinate® rAHF/ (recombinant antihemophilic factor)	Baxter Healthcare (Genetics Institute)	Blood-clotting Factor VIII for the treatment of hemophilia A	Feb 1992
Recombivax-HB® (recombinant hepatitis B vaccine)	Merck	Hepatitis B vaccine for adolescents and high-risk infants; adults; dialysis; pediatrics	Jan 1987 Jan 1987 Jan 1989 June 1993
Refludan® [lepirudin (rDNA) for injection]	Hoechst Marion Roussel	For anticoagulation in patients with heparin-induced thrombocytopenia and associated thomboembolic disease in order to prevent further thromboembolic complications	Mar-98
Regranex® Gel (gel becaplermin)	Ortho-McNeil/ Chiron	Platelet-derived growth factor treatment of diabetic foot ulcers	Dec 1997
Remicade™ (infliximab)	Centocor	Short-term management of moderately to severely active Crohn's disease including those patients with fistula; treatment of patients with rheumatoid arthritis who have had inadequate response to methotrexate alone	Aug 1998 Nov 1999
Renagel® Capsules (sevelamer hydrochlonde)	GelTex Pharmaceuticals/Genzyme	Reduction of serum phosphorus in patients with end-stage renal disease	Nov 1998

Contd...

Appendix 1–Contd...

Product	*Company*	*Application (Use)*	*Approval Date*
ReoPro™ (Abciximab)	Centocor/ Eli Lilly	Reduction of acute blood clot-related complications for high-risk angioplasty patients; reduction of acute blood clot complications for all patients undergoing any coronary intervention; treatment of unstable angina not responding to conventional medical therapy when percutaneous coronary intervention is planned within 24 hours	Dec 1994 Dec 1997
RespiGam® [immune globulin enriched in antibodies against respiratory synctytial virus (RSV)]	Medimmune	Prevention of respiratory synctytial virus in infants under 2 with bronchopulmonary dysplasia or history of prematurity	Jan 1996
Retavase™ reteplase recombinant plasminogen activator)	Centocor	Management of acute myocardial infarction in adults	Oct 1996
Rituxan™ (Rituximab)	IDEC Pharmaceuticals/ Genetech	Treatment of relapsed or refractory low-grade or follicular, CD20-positive B-cell non-Hodgkin's lymphoma	Nov 1997
Roche Amplicor HIV-1 RNA Test	Roche Molecular Systems	*In vitro* nucleic acid amplification test used for patient monitoring and as an aid in management of patients on antiviral therapy for HIV diseases	March 1999

Contd...

Appendix 1–Contd...

Product	*Company*	*Application (Use)*	*Approval Date*
Roferon-A® (recombinant interferon alfa-2a)	Hoffmann-La Roche	Treatment of hairy cell leukemia; AIDS-related Kaposi's sarcoma; chronic phase Philadelphia chromosome positive chronic myelogenous leukemia; hepatitis C	June 1986 Nov 1988 Oct 1995 Nov 1995
Saizen® (recombinant human growth hormone)	Serono Laboratories	Treatment of growth hormone deficiency in children	Oct 1996
Serostim®	Serono Laboratories	Treatment of cachexia (AIDS-wasting)	Aug 1996
Simulect® (basiliximab)	Novartis Pharmaceutical Corporation/Ligand Pharmaceuticals	Prevention of acute rejection episodes in kidney transplant recipients	May 1998
SYNAGIS™ (palivizumab)	MedImmune	Prevention of serious lower respiratory tract disease caused by respiratory syncytial virus (RSV) in pediatric patients at high risk of RSV disease	June 1998
Tamiflu™ (oseltamivir phosphate)	Hoffmann-La Roche/ Gilead Sciences	Treatment of most common strains of influenza (A & B)	Oct 1999
Thyrogen® (thyrotropin alfa for injection)	Genzyme	Adjunctive diagnostic tool for serum thyroglobulin (Tg) testing with or without radioiodine imaging in the follow-up of patients with thyroid cancer	Dec 1998

Contd...

Appendix 1–Contd...

Product	Company	Application (Use)	Approval Date
Targetin® (bexarotene)	Ligand Pharmaceuticals	Treatment of cutaneous manifestations of cutaneous T-cell lymphoma in patients who are refractory to at least one prior systemic therapy	Dec 1999
Tripedia®	Pasteur Mérieux Connaught	Vaccination of infants 2, 4 and 6 months of age and first booster at 15-18 months; primarily for whooping cough	Nov 1992 July 1996
TriHIBit™	Pasteur Mérieux Connaught	Childhood immunization between 15-18 months for acellular pertussis, diphtheria, tetanus and HIB disease	Sept 1996
Ultra-sensitive Amplicor HIV-1 Monitor test	Roche Molecular Systems	Quantitative assay for HIV-1 RNA used to assess a patient's prognosis by measuring changes in plasma HIV-RNA levels during the course of antiviral treatment	March 1997
Venoglobulin-S® (human immune globulin intravenous 5% and 10% solutions)	Alpha Therapeutic	Treatment of primary immunodeficiencies; idiopathic thrombocytopenic purpurea (ITP); kawasaki disease	Nov 1991 Jan 1995
VISTIDE® (cidofovir injection)	Gilead Sciences	Treatment of cytomegalovirus (CMV) retinitis in AIDS patients	June 1997
Vitravene™ (fomivirsen sodium, injectable)	Isis Pharmaceuticals/ CIBA Vision	Treatment of cytomegalovirus (CMV) retinitis in patients with AIDS	Aug 1998

Contd...

Appendix 1–Contd...

Product	*Company*	*Application (Use)*	*Approval Date*
Wellferon® (interferon alfa-n1, lymphoblastoid)	Glaxo Wellcome	Treatment of chronic hepatitis C in patients 18 years of age or older without decompensated liver disease	March 1999
WinRho SDF®	Nabi	Prevention of Rh isoimmunization in pregnant women and the treatment of thrombocytopenic purpurea (TP) (a platelet disorder that can cause uncontrolled bleeding)	March 1995
Zenapax® (Daclizumab)	Hoffmann-La Roche	Humanized monoclonal antibody for prevention of kidney transplant rejection	Dec 1997

Appendix 2: Biotech Company Products Approved by the FDA in 2000

Product Name (Active Ingredient)	*Company(s) (Developer; Marketer)*	*Product Description*	*Indication*	*Approval Date*
Abreva (docosanol 10% cream)	Avanir Pharmaceuticals; SmithKline Beecham	Long-chain alcohol that interferes with viral entry into cells	Topical treatment for recurrent cold sores (herpes simplex infection); OTC medication	July 2000
Acova (formerly Novastan: argatroban)	Texas Biotechnology; SmithKline Beecham	Anticoagulant; synthetic small molecule derived from arginine; acts as direct inhibitor of thrombin	Prevention or treatment of thrombosis in patients with heparin-induced thrombocytopenia (HIT)	June 2000
AndroGel (testosterone)	Unimed Pharmaceuticals (subsidiary of Solvay Pharmaceuticals)	Testosterone	Testosterone replacement therapy in males with testosterone deficiency	Feb 2000
Angiomax (formerly Higulong; bivalirudin)	The Medicines Co. (licensed from Biogen); Innovex	Synthetic thrombin inhibitor based on hirudin (natural anticoagulant secreted by leeches)	Anticoagulant for patients with unstable angina undergoing percutaneous transluminal coronary angioplasty	Dec 2000
CroFab (crotalidae polyvalent immune Fab [ovine])	Protherics; Savage Laboratories	Mixture of 4 different monosepcific antivenins (immunoglobulin fragments produced in sheep)	Management of patients with minimal or moderate North American crotalid envonomation (rattlesnake antivenim)	Oct 2000

Contd...

Appendix 2–Contd...

Product Name (Active Ingredient)	*Company(s) (Developer; Marketer)*	*Product Description*	*Indication*	*Approval Date*
Mylotarg (gemtuzumab ozogamicin)	Celltech Group; Wyeth-Ayerst (AHP)	Humanized anti-CD33 monoclonal antibody, conjugated with calicheamicin (chemotherapy)	Replaced acute myeloid leukemia in CD33+ patients who are 60+ years old and are not candidates for cytotoxic chemotherapy	May 2000
Olux (clobetasol proprinoate 0.05% foam)	Connetics (licensed from Soltec Research Pty.)	High-potency corticosteroid (foam formulation)	Short-term, topical, treatment of moderate-to-severe dermatoses of the scalp	May 2000
Pacis (BCG, live)	BioChem Pharma; UroCor	Live attenuated mycobacteria (Bacillus Calmette-Guerin)	Immunotherapy for bladder cancer	March 2000
Refacto (antihemophilic factor recombinant)	Genetics Institute; Wyeth-Ayerst (AHP) (purchased rights from Pharmacia & Upjohn 8/97)	Recombinant Factor VIII SQ; albumin-free	Hemophilia A; also short-term prophylaxis to reduce frequency of spontaneous bleeding episodes	March 2000
Sarafem (fluoxetine HCl)	Interneuron Pharmaceuticals; Eli Lilly	Synthetic compound (same active ingredient as Prozac) that increases brain serotonin levels	Premenstrual dysphoric disorder	July 2000

Contd...

Appendix 2–Contd...

Product Name (Active Ingredient)	*Company(s) (Developer; Marketer)*	*Product Description*	*Indication*	*Approval Date*
Targretin Gel (bexarotene)	Ligand Pharmaecuticals	Synthetic retinoid analog (selectively activates retinoid X receptors)	Topical treatment of cutaneous lesions in patients with early-stage cutaneous T-cell lymphoma	June 2000
TNKase (tenecte-plase)	Genetech; Boehringer Ingelheim	Bioengineered variant of Activase (tissue plasminogen activator)	Single-bolus thrombolytic agent, to be administered over 5 seconds; treatment of acute myocardial infarction	June 2000
Trisenox (arsenic trioxide)	Cell Therapeutics	Arsenic; induces apopto-sis	Acute promyelocytic leukemia in relapased and refractory patients	Sep 2000
Visicol (sodium phosphate)	InKine Pharmaceutical	Sodium phosphate (tablet formulation)	Cleansing of bowel prior to colonoscopy	Sep 2000
Visudyne (verte-porfin)	QLT PhotoTherapeutics; CIBA Vision	Photodynamic therapy (light-activated drug)	Treatment of wet form of age-related macular degeneration	April 2000
Welchol (formerly CholestaGel; colesevelam HCl)	Genzyme (GelTex Pharmaceuticals); Sankyo; Parke Davis	Non-absorbed polymer that binds bile acids in the intestine (lipid-lowering)	Administered alone or in combination with an HMG-CoA reductase inhibitor (statin), for reducing elevated LDL cholesterol in patients with hyperchloesterolemia	May 2000

Contd...

Appendix 3: Biotech Products Under FDA Review

Product Name	*Company(s) (Developer; Marketer)*	*Product Description*	*Indication (Sought)*	*Submission Type (Date)*
Abarelix Depot	Praecis Pharmaecuticals; Amgen; Sanofi-Synthelabo	Synthetic peptide that acts as a gonadotropin-releasing hormone antagonist	Hormonally response prostate cancer	NDA (Dec 2000)
Acova (a.k.a. Argatroban)	Texas Biotechnology; SmithKline Beecham	Anticoagulant; synthetic small molecule derived from arginine; acts as direct inhibitor of thrombin	Patients who have or who are at risk of developing heparin-induced thrombocytopenia (HIT) and are undergoing percutaneous coronary intervention	Supplemental NDA (Dec 2000)
Alteplase (a.k.a. Activase)	Genentech	Recombinant tPA	To restore function to central venous access devices that have become occluded or blocked	Supplemental BLA (Oct 2000)
Aranesp (darbe-poietin alfa)	Amgen; Kirin	Novel erythropoiesis-stimulating protein (2nd generation EPO)	Patients with chronic renal insufficiency and chronic renal failure	BLA (Dec 1999)

Contd...

Appendix 3–Contd...

Product Name	Company (s) (Developer; Marketer)	Product Description	Indication (Sought)	Submission Type (Date)
Atragen	Aronex Phrmaceuticals	Tretinoin (liposomal formulation of all-trans-retinoic acid)	Patients with acute promyelocytic leukemia for whom therapy with tretinoin is necessary but for whom IV administration is required	NDA (Dec 1998);' Non-approvable letter (Sep 1999); Amendment to NDA (July 2000)

Contd...

Appendix 3–Contd...

Product Name (Active Ingredient)	*Company (s) (Developer; Marketer)*	*Product Description*	*Indication (Sought)*	*Submission Type (Date)*
Bexxar (tositumomab, iodine I 131)	Corixa (Coulter Pharmaceutical); SmithKline Beecham	Murine monoclonal antibody against CD20 antigen on B cells, conjugated to I-131	Patients with relapsed or refractory low-grade or transformed low-grade B-cell non-Hodgkin's lymphoma	BLA (July 1999); FDA requested reorganization of BLA (Aug 1999); BLA re-submission (Sep 2000)
Campath (alemutzumab)	Millennium Pharmaceuticals (LeukoSite); Ilex Oncology; Berlex Laboratories (Schering AG)	Humanized monoclonal antibody against CD52 antigen on T and B cells	Chronic lymphocytic leukemia in patients who have been treated with alkylating agents and who have failed fludabarine therapy	BLA (Dec 1999)
Ceplene (formerly Maxamine; histamine dihydrochloride)	Maxim Pharmaceuticals	H2 receptor against	Adjuvant to interleukin-2 for treating patients with advanced metastatic melanoma with liver metastases	NDA (July 2000)

Contd...

Appendix 3–Contd...

Product Name	*Company (s) (Developer; Marketer)*	*Product Description*	*Indication (Sought)*	*Submission Type (Date)*
Dermagraft	Advanced Tissue Sciences; Sm th & Nephew	Human tissue-engineered replacemnet for dermal layer of skin (viable human dermal fibroblasts cultured on a bioresorbable scaffold)	Wound-healing in diabetic foot ulcers	PMA (Aug 2000)
Dynepo (gene-activated EPO)	Transkaryotic Therapies; Aventis Pharma	Human erythropoietin produced via gene activation (inserts DNA sequences into human cells, thus activating the endogenous human gene to stimulate EPO production)	Anemia in patients with chronic renal failure (both dialysis and non-dialysis patients)	BLA (Aug 2000)
Fabrazyme (agalsidase beta)	Genzyme	Recombinant human alpha-galactosidase A	Enzyme replacement therapy for patients with Fabry diseases	BLA (June 2000)
FluMist	Aviron; Wyeth-Lederle Vaccines (American Home Products)	Attenuated, cold-adapted live virus vaccine (intranasal)	To prevent influenza in children and adults	BLA (Oct 2000)

Contd...

Appendix 3–Contd...

Product Name (Active Ingredient)	*Company (s) (Developer; Marketer)*	*Product Description*	*Indication (Sought)*	*Submission Type (Date)*
GL701	Genelabs Technologies	Adrenal hormone [dehydroepiandrosterone (DHEA)]	Systemic lupus erythematosus	NDA (modular) (May 2000-Sep 2000)
Kineret (anakinra)	Amgen	Recombinant interleukin-1 receptor antagonist	Rheumatoid arthritis	BLA (Dec. 1999)
LeuTech	Palatin Technologies; Mallinckrodt	Radiolabeled monoclonal antibody that binds specifically to white blood cells; for *in viva* imaging of infection sites.	Diagnosis of appendicitis in patients with equivocal signs and symptoms	BLA (Nov 1999)

Contd...

Appendix 3–Contd...

Product Name	*Company (s) (Developer; Marketer)*	*Product Description*	*Indication (Sought)*	*Submission Type (Date)*
Natrecor (nesiritide)	Scios	Recombinant B-type natriuretic peptide	Acute congestive heart failure	NDA (April 98); FDA requested further data (April 1999); Amendment to NDA (Jan 2001)
OP-I Implant	Curls (Creative BioMolecules); Stryker	Recombinant human osteogenic protein-1 in collagen matrix	Bone graft substitute for treating non-union fractures of the Tibia	PMA (modular) (April 1998-June 1999)
Peg-Intron (peginterferon alfa-2b)	Enzon; Schering-Plough	Recombinant interferon alfa-2b modified with polyethylene glycol (PEG) to give it longer-acting properties disease	Chronic hepatitis C virus infection in patients 18 years or older with compensated liver	BLA (Dec 1999)

Contd...

Appendix 3–Contd...

Product Name	*Company (s) (Developer; Marketer)*	*Product Description*	*Indication (Sought)*	*Submission Type (Date)*
Pegasys (peginter-feron alfa-2a)	Hoffmann-La Roche	Recombinant interferon alfa-2a modified with PEG	Chronic hepatitis C virus infection in non-cirrhotic and cirrhotic patients with compensated liver disease	BLA (May 2000)
Relenza (zanamivir)	Biota Holdings; Glaxo Wellcome	Neuramindiase inhibitor	Prevention of influenza A and B in adults	NDA (Sep 2000)
Remicade (infliximab)	Centocor (J&J); Schering-Plough	Chimeric monoclonal antibody to tumor necrosis factor-alpha	Combination therapy with methotrexate for reducing joint damage in patients with rheumatoid arthritis	Supplemental BLA (Oct 1999)
Replagel (agalsidase alfa)	Transkaryotic Therapies; Sumitomo Pharmaceu-ticals	Alpha galactosidase A	Enzyme replacement therapy for Fabry disease	BLA (June 2000)
Symlin (pramlintlde acetate)	Amylin Pharmaceuticals	Synthetic version of human hormone amylin	Adjunctive therapy to insulin for treating people with Type I or II diabetes who use insulin	NDA (Dec 2000)

Contd...

Appendix 3–Contd...

Product Name	*Company (s) (Developer; Marketer)*	*Product Description*	*Indication (Sought)*	*Submission Type (Date)*
Uniprost (a.k.a. UT-15)	United Therapeutics	Analog of natural molecule prostacyclin	Pulmonary arterial hypertension	NDA (modular) (Aug 20Q0 Oct 2000)
Xolair (a.k.a. Anti-IgE; rhuMAb-E25)	Genentech; Tanox; Novartis	Recombinant humanized anti-IgE monoclonal antibody	Allergic asthma and seasonal allergic rhinitis	BLA (June 2000)
Zevalin (ibritumomab tiuextan)	Idec Pharmaceuticals; Schering AG	Murine monoclonal antibody that targets CD20 antigen on B cell surface, conjugated to yttrium-90 (used in conjunction with Rituximab)	Radioimmunotherapy for treating low grade or follicular, relapsed or refractory, CD20-positive, B-cell non-Hodgkin's lymphoma and Rituximab-refractory follicular NHL	BLA (11/00)

Contd...

Appendix 4: Biotechnology Drugs for Cancer Diagnosis and Therapy

Cancer Type	*Disease Name*	*Inherited Cancer Gene*	*Gene Location*
Brain	Neurofibromatosis Type 1	NF1 (Neurofibromatosis gene)	17q
Breast	Hereditary breast/ovarian cancer, type 1 & 2	BRCA 1 & 2 cancer-associated genes)	17q
Colon	Hereditary non-polyposis colon cancer, type 1	hMSH2 (DNA mismatch repair gene)	5q
Eye	Herediatry retinoblastoma	RB1 (Retinoblastoma gene)	13q
Kidney	Hereditary Wilms' tumor	WT1 (Wilms' tumor gene)	11q
Ovary	Hereditary breast/ovarian cancer, type 1 & 2	BRCA 1 & 2 (Breast cancer-associated genes)	17q
Skin	Hereditary melanoma, type 1	CDKN2 (Cyclin-dependent kinase 4 inhibitor)	—

GENETIC TESTING

Polymerase chain reaction (PCR), Single-strand conformation polymorphism (SSCP), Heteroduplex-analysis (HA), Restriction fragment length polymorphism (RFLP), Protein truncation test (PTT), DNA sequencing, Southern blot analysis, Immunohistochemistry, Allele specific oligonucleotide analysis and Denaturing gradient gel electrophoresis (DGGE).

Contd...

Appendix 4–Contd...

Breast Cancer

Cancer Type	Disease Name	Inherited Cancer Gene	Gene Location
Diagnosis (Biotech based)	Genetic testing	1. DNA sequencing: *RRAC Analysis* is a clinically available diagnosis. (FDA approved, product of *Myriad Genetics*) 2. Allele specific oligonucleotide analysis 3. Polymerase chain reaction (PCR) analysis 4. Southern blot analysis	
Therapy (Biotech based)	Antibody therapy	*Herception* is an anti-HER2 monoclonal antibody and now is in the phase III clinical trial. (Product of *Genentech*)	
	Gene therapy	*Adenovirus p53* is a recombinant DNA used for intralesional injection with chemoterpary and now is in the phase I clinical trial. (Fox Chase cancer center)	
	Vaccine therapy	*Theratope* is the synthesized cancer antigens and now is in the phase III clinical trial. (Product of Biomira)	

Prostate Cancer

Cancer Type	Disease Name	Inherited Cancer Gene	Gene Location
Diagnosis (Biotech based)	Genetic testing	1. RadioImmunoassay: *ProstaScint* is a radiolabelled monoclonal antibody-based imaging agent. (FDA approved, product of *Cytogen*) 2. Restriction fragment length polymorphism analysis (FDA approved) 3. Pulsed-field gel electrophoresis	
Therapy (Biotech based)	Antibody therapy	*Herception* is an anti-HER2 monoclonal antibody and now is in the phase II clinical trial.(Product of *Genentech*)	
	Vaccine therapy	*Provenge* is the prostatic acid phosphotase-loaded dendritic cells and is in the phase III clinical trial. (Product of *Dendreon*)	

Index